Essential Practices in Hospice and Palliative Medicine

Fifth Edition

Essential Practices in Hospice and Palliative Medicine
Fifth Edition

UNIPAC 6
ETHICAL AND LEGAL PRACTICE

Elizabeth K. Vig, MD MPH
University of Washington
Seattle, WA

Christina L. Bell, MD PhD
Hawaii Permanente Medical Group
Honolulu, HI

Judith C. Ahronheim, MD MSJ
New York Medical College
Valhalla, NY

Caroline A. Vitale, MD
University of Michigan
VA Ann Arbor Healthcare System
Ann Arbor, MI

Reviewed by
Daniel Fischberg, MD PhD FAAHPM
University of Hawaii
Honolulu, HI

Edited by
Joseph W. Shega, MD
Vitas Healthcare
Miami, FL

Miguel A. Paniagua, MD FACP
University of Pennsylvania
Philadelphia, PA

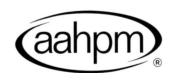

AMERICAN ACADEMY OF
HOSPICE AND PALLIATIVE MEDICINE

8735 W. Higgins Rd., Ste. 300
Chicago, IL 60631
aahpm.org | PalliativeDoctors.org

The information presented and opinions expressed herein are those of the editors and authors and do not necessarily represent the views of the American Academy of Hospice and Palliative Medicine. Any recommendations made by the editors and authors must be weighed against the healthcare provider's own clinical judgment, based on but not limited to such factors as the patient's condition, benefits versus risks of suggested treatment, and comparison with recommendations of pharmaceutical compendia and other medical and palliative care authorities.

Some discussions of pharmacological treatments in *Essential Practices in Hospice and Palliative Medicine* may describe off-label uses of drugs commonly used by hospice and palliative medicine providers. "Good medical practice and the best interests of the patient require that physicians use legally available drugs, biologics, and devices according to their best knowledge and judgment. If physicians use a product for an indication not in the approved labeling, they have the responsibility to be well informed about the product, to base its use on firm scientific rationale and on sound medical evidence, and to maintain records of the product's use and effects. Use of a marketed product in this manner when the intent is the 'practice of medicine' does not require the submission of an Investigational New Drug Application (IND), Investigational Device Exemption (IDE), or review by an Institutional Review Board (IRB). However, the institution at which the product will be used may, under its own authority, require IRB review or other institutional oversight" (US Food and Drug Administration, https://www.fda.gov/RegulatoryInformation/Guidances/ucm126486.htm. Updated January 25, 2016. Accessed May 17, 2017).

Published in the United States by the American Academy of Hospice and Palliative Medicine, 8735 W. Higgins Rd., Ste. 300, Chicago, IL 60631.

© 2017 American Academy of Hospice and Palliative Medicine
First edition published 1997
Second edition published 2003
Third edition published 2008
Fourth edition published 2012

AAHPM Education Staff

Julie Bruno, Director, Education and Learning
Angie Forbes, Manager, Education and Learning
Kemi Ani, Manager, Education and Learning
Angie Tryfonopoulos, Coordinator, Education and Learning

AAHPM Publishing Staff

Jerrod Liveoak, Senior Editorial Manager
Bryan O'Donnell, Managing Editor
Andie Bernard, Assistant Editor
Tim Utesch, Graphic Designer
Jean Iversen, Copy Editor

ISBN 978-1-889296-26-5

Contents

Tables

Figure

Acknowledgments

AAHPM is deeply grateful to all who have participated in the development of this component of the *Essential Practices in Hospice and Palliative Medicine* self-study program. The expertise of the editors, contributors, and reviewers involved in the current and previous editions of the *Essentials* series has ensured the value of its content to our field.

AAHPM extends special thanks to the authors of previous editions of this volume, Ryan R. Nash, MD MA, Leonard J. Nelson, JD LLM, Emily Jaffe, MD MBA, C. Porter Storey Jr., MD FACP FAAHPM, and Carol F. Knight, EdM; the authors of the *UNIPAC 6 amplifire* online learning module, Christina Bell, MD, Britni Lookabaugh, MD, and Beth Popp, MD HMDC FACP FAAHPM; the pharmacist reviewer for this edition of the *Essentials* series, Jennifer Pruskowski, PharmD; and the many professionals who volunteered their time and expertise to review the content and test this program in the field—Joseph Rotella, MD MBA HMDC FAAHM, David Barnard, PhD, Baruch A. Brody, PhD, Ira R. Byock, MD FAAHPM, John W. Finn, MD FAAHPM, Walter B. Forman, MD, Michael E. Frederich, MD FAAHPM, Deon Cox Haley, DO, Gerald H. Holman, MD FAAFP, Timothy J. Keay, MD MA-Theology, Stacie Levine, MD, Neil MacDonald, CM MD FRCPC FRCP, Eli N. Perencevich, DO, Joseph W. Shega, MD, Julia L. Smith, MD, and David Wollner, MD.

Essential Practices in Hospice and Palliative Medicine was originally published in 1998 in six volumes as the *UNIPAC* self-study program. The first four editions of this series, which saw the addition of three new volumes, were created under the leadership of C. Porter Storey Jr., MD FACP FAAHPM, who served as author and editor. AAHPM is proud to acknowledge Dr. Storey's commitment to and leadership of this expansive and critical resource. The Academy's gratitude for his innumerable contributions cannot be overstated.

Continuing Medical Education

Continuing medical education credits are available, and Maintenance of Certification credits may be available, to users who complete the *amplifire* online learning module that has been created for each volume of *Essential Practices in Hospice and Palliative Medicine*, available for purchase from aahpm.org.

Introduction to Ethics

Ethics is the study of right and wrong, good and bad. Ethics assumes that such categories exist, but recognizes that these categories are not always dichotomous. Ethics does not always deal with absolutes; instead it strives to find the better options on the moral gradient.

Ethics is a translational field.[1] Its basic informative disciplines include philosophy, theology, anthropology, history, literature, and the arts (see **Figure 1**). Its applied disciplines include medicine, other health professions, and law. Much like the ideal flow of information in the translational sciences, the flow of ethical discourse is top down and bottom (applied) up. The more applied the field, the louder the voice of the applied disciplines, and vice versa for the theoretical and basic fields. Professionalism, in part, emphasizes the importance of those within the applied field of medicine to have the prominent voice in ethical discourse.

A Brief History of Medical Ethics

Throughout history, systems of healing usually included elements of medical ethics, for example, respect for life, competence, compassion, politeness, and nondiscrimination.[2] The ethical principles outlined in the Hippocratic Oath were widely accepted as the basis for medical ethics for more than 2,500 years. In 1847, the code of ethics developed by the American Medical Association presented medical ethics as not just a set of gentlemanly virtues but also required behaviors, including a clinician's duties to a patient.[3]

Major changes in social, political, economic, medical, and judicial institutions during the 20th century led to widespread concerns about medical ethics and a renewed interest in ethical decision making. No longer could medical ethics be determined solely by the medical profession or the clergy, nor could they remain immune from changes in society.[4]

Figure 1. Ethics as a Translational Field

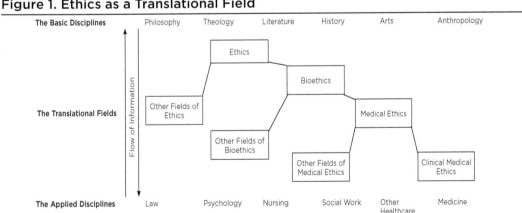

Bioethics as a discipline began in the United States in the 1950s in reaction to medical paternalism,[5] which sometimes jeopardized patients' rights, and the rise of medical technology. During the 1980s many philosophers, religious leaders, and medical ethicists reached consensus on four ethical principles.[6] Two of the principles—beneficence and nonmaleficence—were based on the Hippocratic Oath, but autonomy and justice were new and appeared to contradict more traditional principles in some situations.[4,6] Ethical dilemmas encountered in clinical practice often are discussed in terms of conflicts among these ethical principles. Analyzing ethical dilemmas through application of the ethical principles is one approach, however. Other paradigms also may be useful in analyzing ethical dilemmas (**Table 1**).

A Framework for Approaching Ethical Dilemmas

Clinical Situation

Mr. Baar

Mr. Baar is a 68-year-old veteran with a history of coronary artery disease, peripheral vascular disease, cirrhosis, chronic obstructive pulmonary disease (COPD), and post-traumatic stress disorder. He is admitted to the hospital with a COPD exacerbation. Despite receiving aggressive care in the intensive care unit (ICU), he develops respiratory failure, requiring intubation, decompensation of his liver disease, and worsening of his renal function. He also has hyperactive delirium. After a month of care focused on life prolongation, his condition has not improved. He is estranged from all relatives except for a cousin who lives far away and who is designated as his healthcare agent through a durable power of attorney for health care. The ICU team has spoken to the patient's cousin on multiple occasions. She describes Mr. Baar as a very independent man who managed to live on his own despite his medical problems. She also describes him as a "fighter" who had told her on two different occasions that if anything happened to him, he wanted her to help him live. She understands that his condition remains poor and that the chances of him living independently are very low. During phone calls, she appears to be struggling with balancing his desire to be independent and engaged with the world with his comments about wanting to live. The palliative care team is consulted and asked to "get the Do Not Attempt Resuscitation (DNAR) order."

 How would you approach your conversation with Mr. Baar's cousin? With the primary team?

 What framework could be utilized to organize your thoughts about approaching the ethical aspects of this case prior to making recommendations?

Table 1. Selected Ethical Paradigms

Principle Based

Focuses on the following ethical principles:

- *Beneficence*—Promote patient well-being.
- *Autonomy*—Respect patient self-determination.
- *Nonmaleficence*—Do no harm.
- *Justice*—Protect vulnerable populations and provide fair allocation of resources.

Are conflicts among principles leading to the ethical dilemma?

Virtue Based

Virtues defining the character of a good physician include the following[7]:

- *Fidelity to trust and promise*—honoring the ineradicable trust of the patient-physician relationship
- *Effacement of self-interest*—protecting the patient from exploitation and refraining from using the patient as a means to advance power, prestige, profit, or pleasure
- *Compassion and caring*—exhibiting concern, empathy, and consideration for the patient's plight
- *Intellectual honesty*—knowing when to say "I do not know"
- *Prudence*—deliberating and discerning alternatives in situations of uncertainty and stress.

What values or goals seem to be shared by different stakeholders?

Harms/Benefits

What are the harms and benefits to stakeholders of the different options?

Casuistry

Can responses to previous cases inform the current one?

Professionalism

Professionalism involves the qualities that make a good professional or a good physician. The ways in which a practitioner is true to a standard when honoring established principles, oaths, or examples determines her level of professionalism.

Caring Based

The ethics of caring assume that connections to others are central to what it means to be human. Caring requires empathy and compassion for patients, assuming responsibility for patients by performing actions that meet their needs, and creating an educational environment that fosters caring.[7]

Respect for Personhood

Respect for personhood proposes the following[8]:

- Treatment of patients must reflect the inherent dignity of every person regardless of age, debility, dependence, race, color, creed, etc.
- Actions must reflect the patient's current needs.
- Decisions must value the person and accept human mortality and medical finitude.

All clinicians encounter ethical dilemmas in their work. Ethical dilemmas occur when there is uncertainty or conflict in values among stakeholders. Caring for patients can be stressful for clinicians when ethical dilemmas exist. Familiarity with a framework for thinking about and approaching these dilemmas may reduce clinician distress and burnout.

Different frameworks for thinking about and approaching ethical dilemmas include the four-box approach,[2] Kaldjian's approach,[3] and the CASES approach developed by the VA's National Center for Ethics in Health Care.[4] Although the CASES approach was developed for ethics consultants within the VA system, its five steps can be helpful to others and will be described in **Table 2**.

The first step of the CASES approach, *clarify,* aims to identify whether the dilemma is due to an ethics issue. For example, some dilemmas arise from legal, not ethical, questions. In the case of Mr. Baar, if the question is who should be his legal surrogate decision maker, this is a legal question that would depend on VA or state laws and hospital policies.

In determining if the dilemma is due to ethics, the clinician tries to identify whether there is uncertainty or conflict in values among stakeholders about the right thing to do in a given situation. The medical decision that is being questioned is whether Mr. Baar's status can be changed to Do Not Attempt Resuscitation (DNAR) without his surrogate's consent. The conflict and questioned decision can be put into an ethics question. In this case, the ethics question might be: Given the conflict between the patient's cousin, who believes she should honor her cousin's request to live, and the medical team, who believe that because his chances of recovery are poor and he will not reach his goal of being independent and that he should have a DNAR order, is it ethically appropriate to write a DNAR order without the surrogate's consent? Complex cases sometimes have more than one potential ethics question. For example, in the case of Mr. Baar, the question might not be about whether to write a DNAR order, but whether to transition to comfort care or insert a permanent feeding tube.

Once the ethics question has been formulated, information needed to answer that question is gathered in the second step of the CASES approach, the *assemble* step. As noted in Table 2, there are different types of information that are gathered in this step.

In this step, the relevant medical information is examined. For example, Mr. Baar's condition and chances of recovery would be examined closely. Mr. Baar's preferences would also be examined, as well as his living will. A discussion with his cousin is warranted to learn more about Mr. Baar's life and values and to better understand his desire to live and whether this applied to all situations. It also would be helpful to talk to others who knew him, such as friends, and to the involved clinicians to understand their perspectives.

In cases such as this, it is important to remember that healthcare professionals have much more homogenous beliefs about what they want at the end of life than the general public[5,6,9] (see also Medically Futile or Potentially Inappropriate Treatments on page 29). We might need to remind the medical team that while none of them might want their lives prolonged in Mr. Baar's situation, some patients would want to live in his situation. We would want to look at

Table 2. CASES Approach

Clarify the consultant request.
- Is there an ethical dilemma? Is there uncertainty or conflict in values about the right thing to do?
- What are the stakeholder values that are in conflict?
- What medical decisions are being questioned?
- Construct an ethics question in the format:
  - » Given the conflict between party A's value of X, and party B's value of Y, is it ethically appropriate to do/not do Z?

Assemble the relevant information.
- What information is needed to answer the ethics question?
  - » medical information
  - » patient preferences and interests
  - » other parties' preferences and interests
  - » ethics knowledge (eg, codes of ethics, literature, policies/laws, expert opinion).

Synthesize the information.
- What is the ethical analysis?
  - » What are the consequences for stakeholders of the different options?
  - » What options are ethically acceptable when examined using different ethical paradigms (see Table 1)?
- What are the ethically appropriate options?

Explain the Synthesis.
- Share ethically appropriate options and rationale with others.

Support the consultation process.
- Are there systems-level interventions to prevent similar situations in the future?

Adapted from Ethics Consultation: Responding to Ethics Questions in Health Care, by US Department of Veterans Affairs. Retrieved from http://www.ethics.va.gov/integratedethics/ecc.asp. Accessed May, 30, 2017.

the hospital's informed consent and DNAR policies. Finally, we might want to look at the literature to see what has been written about patients who request life-prolonging care and help resolving conflicts with surrogates.

After gathering all this information, we would proceed to the *synthesize* step. In this step, an ethical analysis of the relevant information is undertaken. One approach to ethical analysis is to examine the case using different ethical paradigms. In Table 1, some different ethical paradigms are presented. Another approach is to think through the consequences of the different options for stakeholders. For example, if a DNAR order is written, what will this mean for Mr. Baar and his autonomy, care, and prognosis; for his cousin and her stress and trust of the medical team; and for the medical team? And does this follow the hospital's policy? After doing our analysis, we could make recommendations about the ethically appropriate options.

After recommendations about the ethically appropriate options are developed, these recommendations and their rationale can be shared with others involved in Mr. Baar's care. This would occur in the *explain* step. Although this step may be more important to ethics consultants than to others applying the CASES approach to ethical dilemmas, it can be helpful for teams caring for patients in challenging situations to have the opportunity to discuss the case together. Others caring for him also might be distressed about the situation. Having an opportunity to discuss and understand the recommendations might help all team members to have a better understanding of the situation, even if they might not agree with the recommendations.

The final step of the CASES approach is *support*. Although it may be more relevant to ethics consultants than to others applying the approach to dilemmas they encounter, support may be helpful to consider. For example, consider the possible recommendations in Mr. Baar's case, that a DNAR order cannot be written over the objections of the patient's cousin. If this situation comes up repeatedly in the ICU, the team might want to consider what interventions would help reduce clinician stress about this issue. They might want to consider whether the current hospital policy needs to be updated. They also might want to develop scheduled team care rounds to discuss challenging cases, or educate providers about the ethically appropriate options for resuscitating patients when chances of recovery are extremely poor. For example, although slow codes are unethical, those running the code can quickly determine that continuing resuscitation efforts are not medically appropriate and stop cardiopulmonary resuscitation.

Ethical Decision Making

The decisions made by terminally ill patients and their clinicians can profoundly affect the life of the patient and family. When clinicians and patients face ethical decisions about emotionally charged issues, such as withholding or withdrawing life-sustaining treatment, the palliative medicine model of care recognizes the importance of shared communication and respect for the multiple and sometimes conflicting needs of clinicians, patients and family members, and interdisciplinary team members. Palliative medicine also acknowledges the intellectual, emotional, and spiritual challenges accompanying ethical decision making for everyone involved in the decision-making process. To arrive at the best decision for a patient and to minimize unnecessary decision-making burden while honoring patient self-determination, an informed consent process using shared decision making should be used. Informed consent gives the opportunity for informed refusal. Patients should be given the opportunity to accept or refuse potentially effective treatments, even if it is not the preferred choice recommended by the provider and seems to conflict with the provider's own values. On the other hand, clinicians are not ethically obligated to provide treatments demanded by the patient or family that are not within the prevailing standards of medical care[10] (see Medically Futile or Potentially Inappropriate Treatments on page 29).

Shared decision making is a way to ensure better informed consent, and it also helps align patient goals and values with available treatments (see **Table 3**). The shared decision-making process is a response to past medical paternalism, when clinicians decided for patients and often acted without adequate communication or opportunity for refusal. Medical paternalism assumed that the physician knew what was best for the patient. In Table 3, shared decision making also is contrasted with informed decision making, in which the physician gives the patient medical information and expects the patient to make a decision on his or her own. Shared decision-making models reflect the fact that physicians and patients have differing spheres of expertise: the physician has knowledge of diseases and their treatments, while the patient has a lifetime of personal experiences and knowledge about their own values and priorities. The goal of shared decision making is to have the best plan for a patient and to ensure their decisions are "informed." Interventions to improve the adoption of shared decision making by healthcare professionals[11] and decision aids for patients[12] have been evaluated by 2014 *Cochrane* reviews but have produced mixed results.

The clinician plays a key role as facilitator in the shared decision making process. In an understandable reaction against paternalism, many clinicians may be reluctant to share their recommendations with patients for fear of overly influencing them and diminishing patient autonomy; however, this reluctance may deprive patients and families of the clinician's expertise and guidance. Clinicians should make recommendations based on their medical knowledge tailored to what they have learned about the patient's values and priorities. Final decisions should be made by patients and their families.

Table 3. Models of Treatment Decision Making

Analytical Stages	Models	Paternalistic	Shared	Informed
Information exchange	Flow	One way (largely)	Two way	One way (largely)
	Direction	Physician → patient	Physician ⟷ patient	Physician → patient
	Type	Medical	Medical and personal	Medical
	Amount	Minimum legally required	All relevant for decision making	All relevant for decision making
Deliberation		Physician alone or with other physicians	Physician and patient (plus potential others)	Patient (plus potential others)
Deciding on treatment to implement		Physicians	Physician and patent	Patient

Reprinted from Social Science & Medicine, 49(5), C Charles, A Gafni, and T Whelan, Decision-making in the physician-patient encounter: revisiting the shared treatment decision making model, 651-661, © 1999, with permission from Elsevier

When patients reach branch points in their medical care in which medical decisions are needed, clinicians need to consider the following:

- What are the elements of informed consent?
- Does the patient have decisional capacity? If so, does he or she want to make the decision? Are there others from whom the patient wants support in decision making?
- If the patient does not have decisional capacity, who is the patient's legal decision maker, surrogate decision maker, or healthcare agent (through a durable power of attorney [DPOA] for health care)?
- How should surrogates make decisions for loved ones?

Clinical Situation

Mrs. Smythe

Mrs. Smythe is a 72-year-old woman who lives independently. A neighbor brings her to her primary care physician because the neighbor has noted that Mrs. Smythe hasn't been out of her house recently. Mrs. Smythe complains of shortness of breath and is admitted to the hospital with pneumonia. She is diagnosed with pneumonia and metastatic lung cancer. She is seen by oncology and agrees to chemotherapy. Her children, who have flown in from out of town to be with her, express concern that her current decision to undergo chemotherapy contradicts previously expressed preferences. They note that she was treated for breast cancer in the past, and, after being told she was cancer free, she had commented that she would never undergo more cancer therapy. They also note that she has a living will stating that she does not want life-sustaining treatments in any of the listed scenarios. They note that she has become more forgetful in the past year. They question whether she agreed to chemotherapy without truly understanding the risks because she was embarrassed to ask clarifying questions and didn't want to offend those taking care of her in the hospital.

 How would you determine whether a true informed consent process took place in the case of Mrs. Smythe?

 What elements comprise the informed consent process?

Informed Consent in Clinical Care

"Informed consent is a process of communication between the healthcare provider or investigator and the patient or research participant that ultimately culminates in the authorization or refusal of a specific intervention or research study."[13] Informed consent is applicable in both clinical and research settings. The goal in both cases is to promote patient autonomy. Interventions to improve informed consent were evaluated in a 2013 *Cochrane* review, which reported that the interventions improved knowledge, but further conclusions were limited by the wide variety of interventions and measures in the studies.[14] (Informed consent for palliative care research is discussed on page 69.)

Informed consent is a process that includes the following elements: disclosure, comprehension, voluntary choice, and authorization.[13] For all planned interventions regardless of intensity, clinicians must first disclose the following information to the patient or the patient's surrogate:

- the patient's diagnosis
- the risks and benefits of performing the proposed procedure
- alternative treatments that may be available
- the risks and benefits of forgoing the proposed treatment.[15]

In determining what information should be shared to allow the patient to make a decision, states operate with different standards. Many states follow the physician-based standard, in which physicians are required to provide information to patients in accordance with the prevailing medical norms. But other states follow the reasonable patient standard, in which physicians are required to provide patients with information that reasonable, prudent patients in the same situation would consider material to make an informed decision.[16]

Comprehension is a vital piece of informed consent. Patients and surrogates must have the capacity to understand the information. Patients and surrogates also must be able to make a voluntary choice. There is no state or federal mandate for signed consent for a procedure, but it is necessary to document these conversations, and it is generally advisable to use institution-specific forms for major procedures. It can be considered unethical to place an IV, draw labs, or change care settings without obtaining a patient's or surrogate's consent before proceeding.[17]

Obtaining adequate informed consent in hospice and palliative care settings may be difficult for many reasons. Many patients are frail, seriously ill, and confused, and have multiple physical, cognitive, emotional, spiritual, and social problems. These conditions make it difficult for them to understand a consent request. Communication strategies, decision aids, and a focus on shared decision making can help improve patients' understanding in the consent process.[12-14]

If a patient has decision-making capacity, informed consent should be obtained from the patient. If a patient is incapacitated, informed consent should be obtained from the legal surrogate. In these cases, efforts should be made to have the patient participate in the decision as much as possible, but the legal surrogate should be the one from whom the informed consent is obtained. On the other hand, patients with mild dementia characterized by short-term memory loss should not reflexively be deemed to lack capacity. Although cases need to be individualized, patients may often be able to participate in the informed consent process. These patients may not necessarily recall the decision they chose, but when the options are explained, they may choose the same consistent option, providing evidence of consistent preferences.

Interventions to improve the adoption of shared decision making by healthcare professionals were evaluated in 2014, but the low quality of evidence limited definitive conclusions.[11] However, the authors suggested that any intervention that actively targets patients, healthcare professionals, or both, is better than none, and that interventions that targeted both patients and clinicians were better than those targeting only patients or clinicians.[11] Decision aids for patients were evaluated by a *Cochrane* review updated in 2014,[12] and it was reported that decision aids improve people's knowledge regarding options, reduce decisional conflict related to feeling uninformed or unclear about values, and improve provider-patient communication. Studies reported mixed effects of decision aids on length of consultation, and more studies are needed to understand the impact of decision aids on adherence, cost effectiveness, and use in low-literacy populations.[12]

In the case of Mrs. Smythe, her children question whether she truly gave informed consent for chemotherapy, because this goes against her previously stated preferences. Further investigation by the medical team reveals that she wants to please her healthcare team and has well-developed social skills. She knows she is in the hospital for pneumonia but does not remember or believe that she has lung cancer. The team begins to question whether she has decisional capacity to consent to chemotherapy.

Determining Decisional Capacity

Patients must have decisional capacity to make their own medical decisions. That is, does the patient have the cognitive abilities to understand the risks, benefits, and alternatives to a proposed treatment? Clinicians are tasked with determining if their patients have this capacity. Decisional capacity can be determined by any clinician. Determinations of capacity by psychiatrists should be reserved for the most difficult situations. Ordinarily this determination can be made by clinicians without the involvement of a court. Of note, clinicians determine if a patient has *decisional capacity* to make a decision, and courts determine if patients are *competent* to make decisions. In most states, patients younger than 18 years are deemed incompetent to make medical decisions with some exceptions (eg, abortions, contraception, substance abuse treatment). In a judicial proceeding, a court may declare that a person is incompetent in business or financial matters and appoint a general guardian, but that person may retain capacity to consent to or refuse medical care.

Several aspects of decisional capacity are important to remember because misconceptions about decisional capacity among clinicians exist.[18] First, capacity is relevant to the decision at hand. Patients with cognitive impairment, for example, may not be able to make complicated decisions about their medical care but may be able to make less complicated decisions. Some individuals with mild dementia may not be able to make complex decisions but may be able to understand the role of a surrogate decision maker and designate someone through a DPOA for health care. Patients with delirium may still be able to make some decisions when their delirium wanes. If a patient has cognitive impairment or active mental illness, this does not automatically indicate that he is unable to make his own decisions.

A patient is presumed to have decision-making capacity unless proven otherwise. It is important to confirm decision-making capacity to ensure the patient has the ability to execute an informed refusal or give informed consent.[19] In medical settings it is the physician's responsibility to determine decision-making capacity. Capacity may change depending on the patient's condition and the complexity of the decision in question. Decision-making capacity is decision specific. The same patient may be able to express a simple value judgment (eg, "I want my son to make decisions for me because I trust him") but not be able to understand the risks, benefits, and alternatives of a complex treatment (eg, aortic valve replacement with lifelong warfarin therapy). To have capacity to make a specific decision, a patient needs to be able to[2,20]

- express insight (express sufficient understanding of relevant information and the implications of various treatment choices)
- make an internally rational choice (a decision that is in accordance with personal values and goals); external rationality standards usually equate to whether a person agrees with a decision
- demonstrate that he or she is not delusional as a consequence of delirium or other psychiatric diseases

- express a static preference (not change his or her mind rapidly based on cognitive difficulties).

In clinical settings, physicians should first assess the patient's mental status and then, if necessary, look for treatable physical conditions that may be interfering with the patient's ability to process information and draw conclusions. Decision-making capacity can be temporarily compromised by conditions such as delirium, metabolic imbalances, severe pain, and life-threatening infections. Decision-making capacity also may fluctuate hour by hour because of high dosages of drugs that may be needed to control symptoms, shifts in levels of consciousness caused by advancing disease, and psychological factors such as the patient's denial of serious illness.[21] Shared decision making with people who have mental health conditions is challenging, and further research[22] on this topic is needed.

Despite the emphasis on a patient's right to make healthcare decisions, studies continue to point to difficulties with assessing decision-making capacity in patients with terminal illness.[23] The method used to determine decision-making capacity may affect the outcome of the assessment. Although some professionals base their decisions about decision-making capacity on cognitive and psychological examination data such as a patient's score on the Mini-Mental State Examination,[24] decision-making capacity may be unrelated to performance on mental status examinations. Instruments such as the Aid to Capacity Evaluation[25] have proved more useful.[26] This tool, with training and examples, is available for download at http://www.jcb. utoronto.ca/tools/documents/ace.pdf.[27]

Alternatively, Dr. Mark Siegler has developed the following questions to assess a patient's decisional capacity (questions used with permission):

1. What's your main medical problem right now?
2. What treatment has been recommended?
3. If you receive this treatment, what will happen?
4. If you don't receive this treatment, what will happen?
5. Why have you decided to/not to receive this treatment?

Other professionals base their determinations of a patient's decisional capacity primarily on daily observations and impressions.[21] Asking patients specific questions about their condition, including diagnosis and prognosis, or using hypothetical case vignettes may be a more valid approach.[28] In any case, family members and other healthcare professionals, particularly those with day-to-day contact with the patient, should be included in the assessment process.

When a patient's decision-making capacity fluctuates or is uncertain, further clarification of decision-making capacity may be necessary if the clinician, the patient or surrogate, and the family disagree on treatment decisions. Whenever possible, consensus in decision making among those who care about the patient should be the goal. When disagreements about treatment occur, the best course of action is to wait until the patient regains decision-making capacity. If the patient's lack of decision-making capacity is likely to continue indefinitely, the designated surrogate has the authority to make decisions, especially if they are in line with the patient's advance directive. In some circumstances a surrogate decision maker can act without following the advance directive. If an advance directive is not available, every effort should be made to ascertain and then apply the patient's previously stated preferences and values.[29] If these are unknown, consider the decisions a reasonable person would make under the patient's circumstances (the best interests standard).[20,30]

Patients who are determined to have decisional capacity may elect not to be overly involved in their decision making. It is ethically appropriate for these patients to delegate decision making to others. As they have aged, some members of the World War II generation have elected to delegate decision making to others. As the Baby Boomer generation ages, it is currently unclear if they will follow this pattern, or remain staunchly in favor of making their own decisions.

In the case of Mrs. Smythe, an evaluation of her cognition reveals that she has capacity to consent to treatment for her pneumonia but does not have capacity to consent to chemotherapy. She is unable to weigh the risks and benefits of this treatment and quickly defers, asking the clinicians to "do what you think is best for me." Since she cannot make the decision about chemotherapy, her medical team must identify her legal surrogate decision maker.

Surrogate Decision Making

When a patient is found to lack the capacity to make a given decision, a surrogate decision maker must be identified. Many states have laws that designate a hierarchy of legal surrogate decision makers. In addition, the Department of Veterans Affairs follows a federal directive delineating a hierarchy of legal surrogate decision makers for veterans cared for within the VA healthcare system. State laws vary in terms of which individuals are on the hierarchical surrogate list. States also vary in how disagreements among multiple legal surrogates, such as a patient's children, are handled. Some states require consensus of all individuals in a category, while other states allow the decision of the majority of individuals in a category to move forward. To find the legal decision maker(s), the clinician starts at the top of the list and goes down until there is one or more people in a category. A list of state laws[31] and additional useful information about surrogate decision making is available on the American Bar Association website.[32]

Beauchamp and Childress have developed qualifications for ethically appropriate surrogates.[33] Their criteria are as follows:

- ability to make reasoned judgments (competence)
- adequate knowledge and information
- emotional stability
- a commitment to the incompetent patient's interest, free of conflicts of interest and free of controlling influence by those who might not act in the patient's best interest.

Returning to the case of Mrs. Smythe, the medical team consults with social work to determine her legal decision maker. Her children have a copy of her living will but do not believe she completed a DPOA for health care. She does not have a legal guardian and is widowed, so according to the law in the state in which she lives, her two children are her legal decision makers. They both have equal decision-making rights. The ultimate authority does not automatically go to the eldest child (though some cultures expect the eldest child to be in the decision-making role). In talking to their mother, her children identify that being comfortable and living as independently as possible continue to be two things that she values. They decide to complete the course of antibiotics in hopes that her dyspnea will improve and agree to discharge her home with hospice services.

In contrast to the case of Mrs. Smythe, when an incapacitated patient has no one to speak for him, decision making becomes more difficult. In 2016, the American Geriatrics Society developed a position statement on ensuring ethical decision making for "unbefriended" adults.[34]

An *unbefriended adult* is defined as a patient who "lacks capacity to make decisions, lacks advance directives, and lacks surrogate decision makers, family, or friends."[34] These vulnerable adults are at risk for treatment delays or prolongation of potentially burdensome treatments due to lack of clear guidance regarding preferences for care. The clinical approach recommended for unbefriended adults includes the following:

- ensuring adequate safeguards for a standard team approach to decision making
- considering nontraditional surrogate decision makers
- conducting systematic capacity assessment
- synthesizing all available evidence, including cultural and ethnic factors in approaching decisions
- preventing adults from becoming unbefriended through proactive identification of at-risk adults and careful assistance in documenting care preferences while capacity is still present.

Though a patient possesses "almost absolute authority" to make his or her own medical decisions, the authority of the surrogate is more circumscribed. The basic role of the surrogate is to make decisions in accordance with the desires of the patient.[35] Ordinarily a surrogate decision maker should apply a "substituted judgment" standard that attempts to mirror the decisions the patient would make under the same circumstances.[35] In other words, if the patient could wake up for 15 minutes and fully understand his or her circumstances, what would he or she tell you to do? It is appropriate for a surrogate to rely on statements in a patient's advance directive and other written and oral statements, but qualitative research suggests that surrogates rarely are chosen for their ability to perform these tasks.[36] In the case of withholding or withdrawing artificial nutrition and hydration (ANH) from incapacitated patients who are not terminally ill, some states may require proof by "clear and convincing" evidence that the patient would have refused ANH.[37] Studies have shown that surrogates accurately predict patient preferences about two-thirds of the time.[38]

If information on the patient's preferences and values is insufficient to apply the substituted judgment standard, it may be permissible for the surrogate to apply the "best interests" standard.[35,39] Depending on the circumstances and legal precedents in the jurisdiction, it may be possible to conclude that continuing life-sustaining treatment is not in the patient's best interests.[35,40] Although ethicists and clinicians expect surrogates to use substituted judgment or a patient's best interests when making decisions, data indicate that many surrogates rely on other factors such as their own best interests or mutual interests of themselves and the patient.[41]

The term *substituted interests*, coined in a 2010 *Journal of the American Medical Association* article, describes a practical approach employed by many experienced palliative medicine physicians.[42] This definition includes physician leadership in listening to the values and wishes of patients, contextualizing medical recommendations appropriately for patients, and offering guidance to surrogates in decision making, but not in such a way that reverts to paternalism (**Table 4**).[42]

Challenging a Surrogate

When a surrogate does not appear to be following a patient's previously stated preferences, efforts by the medical team should attempt to understand this reasoning. In the majority of cases, the surrogate will have a valid reason for this divergence from the patient's stated preferences. For example, the patient may not have anticipated the current situation in his living will. The patient may have stated that he did not want any life-sustaining treatments in his living will but may not have considered the situation of temporary use of these measures while a reversible condition, such as a pneumonia, is being treated. This patient's surrogate may be able to explain why going against the patient's living will, in this situation, is warranted. In some cases, the surrogate may be making decisions based on her own values, not the values of the patient.[41] Although this may seem problematic, patients may grant their loved ones leeway in implementing their preferences, and may allow this divergence to promote their loved one's quality of life.[43-45]

Critical care physicians have identified common approaches in handling disagreements with surrogates surrounding the discontinuation of life support: (a) building trust, (b) educating and informing, (c) providing surrogates more time, (d) adjusting surrogate and physician roles, and (e) highlighting specific values.[46] When mistrust is an issue, physicians endeavor to build a more trusting relationship with the surrogate before readdressing decision making (see *UNIPAC 5*).

When a surrogate's designation or decision is challenged and the matter cannot be resolved, it should be discussed at length to clarify the clinical, biographical, cultural, and quality-of-life issues behind the challenge. Most problems can be resolved in this manner. Occasionally a challenge must be referred to an ethics consultant or committee, but a court rarely is needed.

Table 4. The Substituted Interests Model of Surrogate Decision Making

Step	Sample Conversation Starters and Points
Empathy and connection: Acknowledge stresses of the situation and difficulty of the task and attend to needs of the surrogate.	"It must be very difficult to see your loved one so sick."
Authentic values: Understand the patient as a person. *Values:* Interpersonal, moral, religious, familiar, psychological. *Directives:* Substantive treatment preferences and process considerations, such as who should decide and how.	"Tell us about your loved one." "Has anyone else in the family ever experienced a situation like this?"
Clinical data: Share understanding of the patient's clinical circumstances and prognosis.	"All of that is important for us to know as we face the current situation." "Here is what is wrong…" "This is what is likely to happen…"
Substituted interests: Determine what the patient's real interests are, given the patient's values and circumstances.	"Knowing your loved one, what do you think would be most important for him right now? Avoiding pain? Having family members here?"
Clinical judgment: Share understanding of the options and offer recommendations based on clinical experience tailored to the particular patient's real interests.	"Here's what could be done." "This is what we would recommend, based on what we know and what you've told us about your loved one."
Best judgment for the patient: Best path to promote the good of the patient as a unique person, in the context of his relationships, authentic values, known wishes, and real interests, given the circumstances and options	"Knowing your loved one, does our recommendation seem right for him? Do you think another plan would be better, given his values, preferences, and relationships?"

Disagreement Among Members of the Interdisciplinary Team

Because hospice and palliative care attempts to meet a patient's physical, emotional, spiritual, and social needs, the skills and resources of an entire interdisciplinary team are needed. As with any group, differences of opinion are bound to occur among members of the team. In fact, they are an expected part of the creative process of working together. When skillfully managed by a group facilitator, differences can usually be resolved in a manner that results in better patient care and professional growth for all concerned. On occasion, differences cannot be resolved by discussion. If consultation with an ethics consultant or counseling does not resolve the problem, other alternatives to ensure continued effective team dynamics may need to be employed (see *UNIPAC 5* for more information on effective teamwork and communication).

Withdrawal of a Healthcare Professional or Institution

Clinicians with moral or religious objections to providing or withdrawing treatments (such as those of Orthodox Jewish faith[47,48]) demanded by a patient or surrogate must communicate these concerns to the patient or surrogate and arrange for the patient's transfer to another physician, if necessary and feasible. If another member of the team has moral or religious objections to a decision, the institution should honor a request for removal from the case when appropriate, if necessary and feasible. In some areas, hospice and palliative care programs may need to develop policies regarding physician-assisted dying and communicate them openly to associated physicians, prospective patients, and family members. Ethics consultation may help team members better understand and communicate about difficult decisions.

A federal statute known as the Church Amendment supports the rights of healthcare providers to conscientiously refuse to participate in a "program or activity [that] would be contrary to his religious beliefs or moral convictions."[49] Violations of these laws are to be reported to the Office of Civil Rights Enforcement.[50] Those invoking conscience protection may not be doing so only to protect themselves from being involved in an action they believe to be morally wrong. They may be attempting to protect the patient from an action they believe may be harmful, so discussion with staff regarding the burdens and benefits of treatments can be fruitful.

When a patient or surrogate is adamant about obtaining treatments the program cannot ethically provide, as a last resort, the patient can be discharged or transferred to another institution. If a case requires transfer to another provider or institution, a referral to the institution's ethics committee and legal department should be made (see Medically Futile or Potentially Inappropriate Treatments on page 29). In these difficult situations, clinicians need to ensure that patients and families do not feel abandoned by the medical system.

Selected Ethics Topics in Hospice and Palliative Care

Advance Care Planning

Advance care planning is a process whereby individuals think about their values and care preferences, consider what types of care they would and would not want in the future in different medical situations, and discuss their preferences with their loved ones and clinicians. As part of this process, individuals also can identify who should make their medical decisions if they are unable to in the future. As part of advance care planning, people can designate a healthcare agent through a durable power of attorney (DPOA) for health care. They also can document their care preferences in a living will or other instructional directive. In 2016, Medicare began to reimburse clinicians for engaging in advance care planning discussions with their patients. Several advance care planning materials, some with sample directives, are available online (see **Table 5**).

The Patient Self-Determination Act (PSDA), federal legislation enacted in 1990, requires institutional healthcare providers who participate in Medicare and Medicaid programs to provide patients with information about advance directives.[51] The PSDA also requires healthcare providers to document in the medical record whether the patient has executed an advance directive.[35]

Advance directives can either provide instructions on care decisions in the event a patient reaches a specified severity of illness or disability (a living will), or name a proxy or surrogate to make decisions if the patient is not able to do so (a medical power of attorney). These directives are distinct from physicians' orders (do not attempt resuscitation [DNAR] orders or physician orders for life-sustaining treatment [POLST]).

Table 5. Advance Care Planning Resources

- www.nia.nih.gov/health/publication/advance-care-planning
- www.prepareforyourcare.org
- www.americanbar.org/groups/law_aging/resources/health_care_decision_making/consumer_s_toolkit_for_health_care_advance_planning.html
- www.acpdecisions.org
- www.theconversationproject.org
- www.compassionandchoices.org/eolc-tools/
- www.elderguru.com/download-the-your-life-your-choices-planning-for-future-medical-decisions-workbook
- www.agingwithdignity.org

Advance and Instructional Directives

Instructive directives are completed by a person with decision-making capacity and help guide care when the patient loses the capacity to make healthcare decisions. Common examples of instructive directives include living wills, Natural Death Act documents, and medical directives.

All states have adopted laws that provide a framework that permits residents to execute an advance directive to provide guidance in the event that the individual loses decisional capacity in the future.[35] Instructive directives often state the patient's wishes regarding life-sustaining treatment in various clinical situations; these directives are usually activated when a patient loses decision-making capacity. Patients with decision-making capacity have the right to refuse any treatment, and instructive directives extend that right when decision-making capacity is compromised. A clinician's responsibility is to honor the intent of a patient's advance directive and attempt to ensure the care plan can reasonably meet its goals. After consultation with the patient or surrogate, family, and others involved, appropriate physician orders should be written that are consistent with the patient's advance directive. If the patient has decision-making capacity, the advance directive is not operative, and the clinician must obtain informed consent from the patient.[35]

Because advance directives cannot predict every potentiality, they usually serve only as a general guide based on overarching value and goal judgments (eg, "I am willing to accept great burden to prolong my life"). A decision in conflict with the patient's advance directive should be considered when the medical facts are not predicted by the advance directive or when the surrogate believes such a decision is more consistent with the patient's values and makes medical sense. For example, a patient may have completed an advance directive stating that he would not want any life-sustaining treatments at the end of life. His wife, who is his legal decision maker, may decide that he is not terminally ill and would want aggressive treatment for a heart attack. The clinician or other members of the medical team should spend time with the patient's legal decision maker to better understand their rationale for their decision making.

Advance directives can be difficult to understand and complete (the average reading level required for official state directives in the United States is nearly 12th-grade level[52]), even for clinicians. Most instructive directives are ambiguous and lack specific directions. Misunderstanding of standard advance directives and what they mean remains exceedingly common.[53] Although directives often refer to "heroic life-prolonging measures," such measures rarely are defined. Even with the help of computer-based learning aids, clinician confidence in these directives is not high.[54] Many instructive directives fail to state when specific measures should be withheld or withdrawn in the context of an incurable or terminal illness.[55] The majority of patients, even those with progressive cognitive impairment[56] or brain tumors,[57] do not complete these directives. This may explain why they are not always honored and do not appear to affect the cost of terminal admissions of cancer patients.[58]

Typically, state laws absolve clinicians from liability when the clinician follows the instructions in a validly executed advance directive. If the clinician feels that he or she is unable to follow the patient's clearly stated wishes because of his or her personal views or values, the patient can be transferred to the care of another clinician who is willing to comply with the instructions in the directive (see Withdrawal of a Healthcare Professional or Institution on page 17). Ethics or legal consultation should be considered in difficult cases.

Proxy Directives: Designation of Surrogate Decision Makers

If a patient becomes incapacitated, treatment decisions may be made by a proxy or surrogate decision maker. Most states have adopted laws that permit a legally competent individual to execute a document authorizing a surrogate to make healthcare decisions on the individual's behalf, only after that patient loses decision-making capacity. As mentioned throughout this book, these documents are sometimes referred to as DPOA for health care. It is becoming more common to combine a surrogate appointment with an instructive advance directive (eg, *Five Wishes* document). Though some state statutes specifically authorize proxies to make decisions to withhold or withdraw life-sustaining treatment, other state statutes limit the authority of a surrogate, setting standards of evidence required for certain decisions in that regard.[35]

Even if there is an advance directive, its instructions are often insufficient to cover every potential situation. Designation of a surrogate is always recommended. A surrogate appointment that names a decision maker who knows the patient well and understands the spirit of the instructive directive can be an invaluable aid when caring for a person at the end of life. A surrogate appointment is particularly important in certain circumstances, such as a patient naming someone other than a legal spouse to act as his or her surrogate. A proxy also is important when disagreements among family members cannot be resolved or when family members are unavailable or nonexistent.

When the patient is incapacitated and there is no surrogate or guardian with authority to make a medical decision, many states have statutes designating the patient's spouse, then adult children, then parents or siblings to act as the patient's surrogate decision maker.[31,35] In the absence of such a statute, it may be appropriate to presume that close family members who know the patient well have decision-making authority.[35] When there is a lack of consensus among family members regarding the preferred course of treatment and no agreement on a single surrogate, an application may be made to a court to designate one.[35] In the case of an incapacitated patient with no surrogate, no guardian with authority to make medical decisions, and no family, court designation of a surrogate may be necessary (see discussion of unbefriended adults on page 14). Sometimes a patient may have indicated to the treating physician that a person who may not be legally recognized as family by state or federal law act as a surrogate when the patient becomes incapacitated. It may be appropriate in some cases (eg, domestic partners, friends, or other persons with clear interest) for the physician to accept this designation.[35] Neither the patient's physician nor members of an interdisciplinary care team should serve as a patient's surrogate decision maker.

Advance Directives in Hospice and Palliative Care

Completing an advance directive and appointing a proxy can be helpful measures for documenting a patient's preferences and ensuring that his or her wishes are respected in the future. Education and counseling related to treatment choices should precede completion of an advance directive.[59] Periodic reviews of advance directives are particularly important in hospice and palliative care and should be part of the ongoing dialogue between patients and clinicians. As patients deal with debility and chronic illness or are approaching the end of life, they have a better understanding of how they want to live and their fears. Healthcare providers may be better able to anticipate the clinical course. It is important to recognize that serious illness is a dynamic process, and goals of care should be readdressed with each setting and condition change.

Revisiting an advance directive in the setting of a serious or terminal illness can offer rewarding opportunities for exploring several issues, including the patient and family's changing expectations about goals of care, the outcomes of end-of-life care, the patient's values and beliefs about dying and death, and the patient's wishes for specific treatments when decision-making capacity is diminished.[60]

The skill of discussing advance directives must be practiced and honed over time.[61] When patients with serious or life-threatening illnesses are extremely anxious about the thought of dying, discussions about advance directives initiated at the wrong time or in an insensitive manner may lead the patient to become more fearful and less trusting of healthcare providers.

Programs providing end-of-life care should ensure that all appropriate patient records accompany patients from one care setting to another. In addition, hospice and palliative care programs and affiliated clinicians should consider working with local healthcare facilities and emergency medical services systems to develop policies such as POLST that protect identified patients from unwanted resuscitation efforts. It is notable that since 2014, documentation of a discussion of hospice patients' treatment preferences as well as patients' beliefs and values are quality measures that hospices are required to report to Medicare with each hospice admission and discharge (see *UNIPAC 1*).

Outcomes of Advance Care Planning and Advance Directives

What are the known outcomes of advance care planning and completing advance directives? A recent systemic review and meta-analysis examined the efficacy of advance care planning.[62] The authors included 55 trials. Successful interventions focused on completing directives and communicating about end-of-life preferences. More intervention subjects completed advance care directives (odds ratio 3.26) and communicated their preferences about end-of-life care (odds ratio 2.48) than patients in the usual care groups. When communication occurred, there was also improved concordance between patient preferences and the care they received (odds ratio 4.66).

A paper published with data from the large Health and Retirement Study noted that the majority of directives outline preferences to limit care, but 2% of participants wanted "all care possible."[9] The investigators found that more than 90% of those who wanted limited or comfort care in their directives received this type of care prior to death. In a second study, advance directives specifying limitations in end-of-life care were associated with significantly lower levels of Medicare spending, lower likelihood of in-hospital death, and higher use of hospice care in regions characterized by higher levels of end-of-life spending but not in other regions.[63]

Physician Orders

Do Not Resuscitate (or Attempt Resuscitation) Orders

Cardiopulmonary resuscitation (CPR) was developed for selective use on acutely ill patients or victims of acute insults such as drowning, electrical shock, or anesthetic accidents. Over time, hospital resuscitation protocols changed, eventually requiring CPR for all patients experiencing cardiac arrest regardless of underlying illness.[64,65] In fact, resuscitation is the default standard of care unless a DNAR order is in the chart.[66]

Different terms are used when referring to the orders used to forgo CPR. Most clinicians are familiar with the older term, *Do Not Resuscitate,* which has widespread use. Some believe that DNAR is a more accurate term. They argue that the latter term implies that CPR will be attempted but is not a guarantee of successful resuscitation. Others advocate for the term Allow Natural Death. Breault has published a piece in which he discusses the pros and cons of using these three terms.[292] In this book, the term DNAR is used.

Several states have adopted statutes governing DNAR orders.[35] The primary purpose of these statutes is to provide protection to physicians to write DNAR orders and to implement the right of patients to refuse CPR.[35] These statutes vary from state to state, so physicians should follow hospital policy on DNAR orders to ensure compliance with state law.[35]

Rates of survival after CPR vary by patient population. Patients may opt to receive CPR because they believe that survival from CPR is quite high. In one study, patients estimated their CPR survival to be over 60%, while their actual survival was 17%.[67] Factors that lower the chances of survival include older age, functional status, malignancy, and comorbidities.[68] In a large survey, only 3.9% of patients who experienced a cardiopulmonary arrest in the intensive care unit (ICU) were discharged home from the hospital.[69] In a 2015 study of hospitalized patients receiving dialysis who were resuscitated, 21.9% survived to hospital discharge, but the median postdischarge survival was 5 months.[70] A meta-analysis of CPR outcomes for patients with cancer found that the percentage of patients who survive until hospital discharge has increased.[71] Survival of those with metastatic disease overall was 5.6%, compared to a 9.5% survival of those with localized disease. The overall survival rate for patients in an ICU was 2.2%, compared to 10% for those who were discharged from the ICU. Few studies have examined the neurological condition of patients who have survived CPR.

The circumstances in which physicians can ethically make choices on behalf of patients without their consent are continually debated.[64] Physicians often refrain from offering treatments that clearly offer no benefit, and some believe CPR for dying patients falls under this category.[72] Others believe DNAR orders should always be discussed with patients and family members.[73] DNAR issues vary from state to state.[74] In states such as New York, consent to CPR is presumed unless a patient (or legally defined surrogate) explicitly refuses it or unless it is "medically futile," a difficult situation to define. In most cases, CPR is not sound medical practice for patients with terminal illness or those who are irreversibly comatose. A physician's DNAR order should be based on either a patient or surrogate's request or a medical judgment that the patient is dying from a primary disease or injury for which CPR would either be ineffective or for which the burdens of such treatment would outweigh the potential benefits.

Issues Related to DNAR Orders

When curative life-prolonging treatments are no longer appropriate, discussing CPR within the context of changing the goals of care is likely to benefit the patient and family. When engaging in a conversation about end-of-life care preferences, it is better to start the discussion by focusing on the patient's preferred goals of care than on their code status. Of note, many patients find it easier to discuss general quality-of-life considerations than specific medical interventions. After the goals are established, it may then be appropriate to discuss resuscitation. When a healthcare provider understands a patient's values, he or she will be better able to guide the patient through appropriate use of medical technology. If the goals are clearly to pursue life-prolonging care in any situation, then it may not be appropriate to discuss the option of not providing CPR. Alternatively, a patient may want efforts to prolong his life up to the point of death, but may not want to be resuscitated. Because these preferences may not seem compatible to some clinicians, documenting the conversation and patient's rationale for his preferences can be helpful to those caring for the patient in the future and to the patient, who will not have to repeat and explain his preferences to each new clinician involved in his care. The process of shared decision making provides clinicians with opportunities to explore CPR with patients and family members in terms of the goals of care. Race or ethnicity and uncontrolled pain also may be important factors.[75,76] Clinicians may want to include the following in code status discussions[77-79]:

- the resuscitation procedure itself
- probable outcomes when the procedure is applied to frail, terminally ill patients
- interventions that are not automatically withheld when a DNAR order is written (ie, antibiotics, artificial nutrition and hydration [ANH], ventilators, possible transfer to an ICU)
- continued provision of pain and symptom control measures
- continued provision of supportive care
- possibility of changing the decision at any time, if appropriate
- benefit of identifying a surrogate decision maker.

When the potential burdens of CPR far outweigh potential benefits, it is appropriate for the clinician to recommend against CPR and emphasize the available disease-directed and palliative treatments that would be more beneficial. If a patient, surrogate, or family member insists on CPR, even when the clinician believes it is inappropriate, members of an interdisciplinary team should work with all parties to uncover and discuss relevant biographical, clinical, and cultural facts.

In some cases, reluctance to forgo CPR may be based on misconceptions about the CPR procedure and the ramifications of a DNAR order (**Table 6**). In other cases, cultural, ethnic, or religious barriers may influence a patient or family's decision making and should be elicited and respected by the health care team.

Healthcare providers often are stressed when families of patients near the end of life insist on CPR or other invasive interventions "in hopes of a miracle."[80] There is evidence that end-of-life outcomes improve with the provision of spiritual support from medical teams and with a proactive approach to medical decision making that values statements given by patients and family members.[81] The following issues should be explored when terminally ill patients, surrogates, or family members continue to insist on near-futile CPR:

- affirmation that a DNAR order is not mandated for hospice and palliative care patients
- patient and family expectations
- goals of hospice and palliative care
- services offered by a particular hospice and palliative care program
- recognition that hospice or palliative care inpatient units may not be equipped to provide resuscitation efforts
- honest prognostication with or without the intervention
- evidence that documentation of a DNAR order, even before surgery, has not been associated with increased mortality[82]
- the impact of such resuscitation efforts on the team and perhaps some advance discussion about the duration of resuscitative efforts on such patients.[83]

Table 6. Misconceptions About CPR and DNAR Orders

CPR is a benign procedure with no potential risks or burdens.

CPR always restores life and restores it to its previous level.

DNAR orders mean that
- death is imminent or the DNAR order will somehow cause death to become imminent
- the patient will be ignored and not receive other curative treatments, particularly in an acute care facility, if inpatient care is required
- nothing will be done to ensure the patient's comfort when the patient actively begins to die
- pain and symptom control measures will cease
- supportive care will end
- the patient is ready and willing to die.

Careful inquiry into the patient or family's reasons for insisting on the provision of CPR may reveal misconceptions about CPR or important grief-related issues that need to be addressed. When a patient or family acknowledges that they are waiting for a miracle to occur, clinicians may want to follow the recommendations made by Delisser.[80] In some rare instances, performing CPR in a futile situation may actually be in the family's best interests.[84]

Family Observation of Cardiopulmonary Resuscitation

In the interest of patient- and family-centered care, some hospitals are moving toward open visiting hours and family areas in or adjacent to patient rooms.[85] This trend increases the likelihood of family or friends observing resuscitation efforts.[86] Advocates want to give families the option of being present during CPR attempts. A recent multicenter randomized trial in France found worse outcomes (more posttraumatic stress disorder, anxiety, and depression) in family members who had not witnessed their loved one's CPR attempt compared to the family members who had witnessed CPR.[87] To avoid undue burden or unethical coercive practice, organizations may want to consider instituting policies that address the following:

- If offered, observing a resuscitation must be voluntary.
- Patient privacy is respected as much as possible (with obvious challenges in doing so).
- A team member who is not involved in the resuscitation effort must actively educate and contextualize the events and actions taking place.
- Counseling and education before and after the event are the expected norm.
- Observation should never be used as a manipulative or coercive method to educate and contextualize the events and actions taken.

Physician Orders for Life-Sustaining Treatments in the Outpatient Setting

When patients, surrogates, or family members call 911 for emergency medical services (EMS), they should expect full resuscitation efforts and transportation to the nearest emergency department unless clearly communicated otherwise. Unless organizations have developed interagency agreements that clarify the role of EMS personnel, CPR likely will be initiated. Clinicians associated with hospice and palliative care programs should become familiar with the organization's written policies on CPR and DNAR orders. Certain states have developed DNAR orders for outpatients. These forms have different names, such as POLST (physician orders for life-sustaining treatment), MOLST (medical orders for life-sustaining treatment), and MOST (medical orders for scope of treatment). Some states have authorized official bracelets or neck pendants to notify emergency personnel to not attempt resuscitation in the event a patient collapses in a public place.

The POLST form was developed in Oregon to honor a patient's DNAR preferences in the outpatient setting and to convey the preferences of skilled nursing home residents when they were transferred to the hospital. The brightly colored POLST form turns a patient's wishes concerning end-of-life treatment as expressed in the course of a conversation with a physician into a medical order with specific treatment instructions. The form is filled out based on the patient's current condition and usually has four sections. The first section addresses the patient's code status. The second section outlines the overall goals of care, ranging from comfort care, to limited care in a hospital, to aggressive life-prolonging care delivered in an ICU setting. The third and fourth sections identify preferences about the use of antibiotics and feeding tubes. The form is signed by the treating physician and the patient or the patient's surrogate. The original copy is given to the patient and should accompany him when he transfers between healthcare settings. A copy is retained in the medical record. Oregon has started a state-wide registry to make POLST preferences available if the original forms are not (see www.orpolstregistry.org). Healthcare workers and emergency responders are required to comply with POLST orders. Some laws provide that a POLST order overrides conflicting instructions in advance directives and decisions by a proxy.

The POLST program, when implemented as envisioned, is consistent with palliative medicine's desire to enhance quality of care and expression of patient wishes across transitions in care. In addition, it helps ensure that physicians are involved in advance care planning and medical decision making. This is a particular concern because many advance directives or living wills are enacted without physician input and without clear information on the disease, prognosis, and expectations. Nonphysician-involved advance directives in some circumstances may be viewed as uninformed or misinformed consent. POLST has been used in hospitals, nursing homes, outpatient geriatric care programs, doctors' offices, and other care settings.

Studies have investigated the use of POLST forms and were recently reviewed.[88] This systematic review found that POLST forms are used more often by white than nonwhite patients, and that nonwhite patients have orders for more aggressive care. One-third of patients overall had preferences for the least aggressive care options (DNAR, comfort measures, antibiotics for comfort, and no artificial nutrition). The review concluded that treatments received "are largely consistent with orders."[88] High rates of consistency were found between patients having DNAR orders and not being resuscitated, and for antibiotic and feeding tube use. As more states adopt their own versions of the POLST form, more data may become available about their overall effectiveness at promoting patient end-of-life preferences across sites of care.

Symptom Management and Principle of Double Effect

Although most pain experienced by terminally ill patients can be adequately controlled using readily available medications and simple techniques, the question remains: Why do so many seriously ill and dying patients continue to experience uncontrolled pain? Several barriers to adequate pain management have been identified on the part of clinicians, patients, and the wider healthcare system. Physicians (even oncologists) report poor training in pain assessment and control.[89] Patients and families often fear addiction or underreport pain, and the healthcare system has established barriers to distributing pain medication.[90,91] (For more in-depth discussion on pain management, refer to *UNIPAC 3*.)

Ethical issues arise in pain management.[92] When caring for palliative care patients, some physicians and nurses may be concerned about the pain medications hastening the patient's death, for example. The principle of double effect has been used to justify practices where there are potentially both good and bad effects (see Principle of Double Effect sidebar below). Some, however, have questioned the universal uptake of this principle in palliative care.[93]

The principle of double effect is an alternative to the benefit-burden ethical framework. This principle emphasizes the intentions of the clinician. According to this view, if the clinician's intent is to relieve pain, prescribing additional opioids is morally acceptable even when the drugs may theoretically shorten a patient's life.

The principle of double effect has been endorsed by the Catholic Church and other organizations. It can be misinterpreted to suggest that opioids should be withheld from a patient with terminal illness until the clinician is ready for the patient to die. There is, however, no evidence that carefully titrated dosages of opioids shorten the lives of terminally ill patients. In fact, many hospice and palliative care clinicians have observed that prescribing dosages of an opioid sufficient to relieve pain and dyspnea can improve activity levels, quality of life,[94] and perhaps even survival.[95]

Principle of Double Effect

Although it has been criticized in recent years, the principle of double effect has had a significant role in the Catholic medico-ethical tradition and has also influenced criminal law.[96] The principle is still used in both Catholic and secular bioethics. It validates the use of treatments that are honestly intended to relieve suffering or restore health even if the intervention has potential untoward effects such as shortening a patient's life. The four elements of this principle are:

- The good effect has to be intended (eg, relieving pain or dyspnea).
- The bad effect can be foreseen but not intended (could possibly shorten life but is not the intent).
- The bad effect cannot be the means to the good effect (cannot end the patient's life to relieve the pain).
- The symptom must be severe enough to warrant taking risks (known as proportionality).

Under the principle of double effect, if the clinician's intent is to relieve dyspnea, prescribing additional opioids is morally and legally acceptable even when the drugs also may theoretically shorten the patient's life.

On the other hand, administering a lethal bolus injection of opioids that results in immediate death could be the basis for a homicide prosecution even if the injection is administered at the request of a patient or surrogate decision maker. Some states have recognized the principle of double effect by enacting statutes that provide immunity from professional discipline or criminal prosecution for clinicians who prescribe drugs that are adequate to control "intractable pain." However, this statutory protection may be unnecessary as no medical research has determined that appropriate use of opioids hastens death in patients receiving palliative care. Furthermore, the legal protection afforded under the principle of double effect is congruent with the ethical requirement that the potential positive effect must be honestly intended and proportionate to the uncertain negative effect. Thus, clinicians who administer opioids to terminally ill patients with the informed consent of the patients or surrogates and in accordance with the prevailing standards of medical care for the primary purpose of relieving pain and suffering generally are not subject to criminal or civil liability even if the opioids arguably theoretically hasten death.

The best legal protection is to use medically appropriate pain and symptom management principles and to carefully document the reasons for the dose increments chosen. Dose increments should also be kept in line with established principles of dose escalation and adjustment.

Medically Futile or Potentially Inappropriate Treatments

Clinical Situation

Mr. Bautista

Mr. Bautista is a 98-year-old skilled nursing home resident with multiple medical problems, including moderate dementia, who is transferred to the hospital with sepsis due to pneumonia. He is admitted to the ICU, where he is intubated and receives care focused on life prolongation. He never completed a living will but designated his only son as his healthcare agent through a DPOA for health care. His son reports that because of his culture (he is from the Philippines) and religion (Catholic), it is not appropriate for him to pursue comfort care for his father. During the next 2 weeks, Mr. Bautista cannot be weaned from the ventilator. His renal function deteriorates. Mr. Bautista's son requests that his father receive a tracheostomy and begin dialysis. The team caring for Mr. Bautista believes that his situation is futile, and begins to question his son's motives for keeping his father alive.

? What aspects of this case may be contributing to the team's beliefs that the treatments the son is requesting may be futile?

? Does the case meet accepted standards for qualitative futility?

? What factors might be driving the son's decisions and preferences?

Rising healthcare costs, increased attention on delivering high-quality care that focuses on the patient experience,[97] along with the growth of palliative care may be placing more pressure on clinicians to withhold or withdraw treatments that offer no real hope or benefit to patients. Although decisions about which treatments to offer and which treatments to withhold or withdraw often are framed in terms of medical futility (see Futile Treatments sidebar below), developing a universally accepted, clinically useful definition of medical futility has proved an elusive task. Nevertheless, society's growing awareness of the limitations of modern therapies has contributed to widespread acceptance of the following statements:

- The existence of a medical therapy does not mandate its use.
- Doing everything possible is not always beneficial to the patient or aligned with the patient's achievable goals and wishes.
- Regardless of treatment, patients with advanced malignancies, end-stage organ failure, and other terminal conditions will eventually die of the disease or related complications.
- Decisions about treatment should be guided by medical indications, a determination of the treatment's likely benefits and potential burdens (physical, psychosocial, financial, and spiritual), and the patient's goals of care.

"Futile" Treatments[98]

In the circumstance that no evidence shows that a specific treatment desired by the patient will provide any medical benefit, the clinician is not ethically obliged to provide such treatment (although the clinician should be aware of any relevant state law). The clinician need not provide an effort at resuscitation that cannot conceivably restore circulation and breathing, but he or she should help the family to understand and accept this reality. The more common and much more difficult circumstance occurs when treatment offers some small prospect of benefit at a great burden of suffering, but the patient or family nevertheless desires it. If the clinician and patient (or appropriate surrogate) cannot agree on how to proceed, there is no easy, automatic solution. Consultation with learned colleagues or an ethics consultation may be helpful in ascertaining what interventions have a reasonable balance of burden and benefit. Timely transfer of care to another clinician who is willing to pursue the patient's preference may resolve the problem. Infrequently, resorting to the courts may be necessary. Some jurisdictions have specific processes and standards for allowing these unilateral decisions.

Making Determinations of Medical Futility

Most clinicians have some commonsense understanding of the concept of medical futility but, when pushed to explain its exact meaning, may respond, "I can't define it, but I know it when I see it."[99] Some treatments offer so little prospect of benefit that it seems useless to offer them.

In such cases clinicians may be reluctant to discuss these types of treatments with patients or families, believing that the discussion would serve no purpose.[72]

Difficulties regarding medical futility are partly attributable to varying definitions. Schneiderman, Jecker, and Jonsen defined medical futility on quantitative and qualitative grounds.[100] If an intervention has a chance of providing benefit but has failed to do so in the last 100 cases, they contend it is quantitatively medically futile (less than a 1% chance of benefit). A treatment is qualitatively futile when it is perceived that the burdens outweigh the benefits of the treatment. Qualitative futility often is considered if a technology is perceived as merely maintaining a patient in a state of permanent unconsciousness (ie, a persistent vegetative state) or in a state that continues to require management in an ICU with no hope of benefit other than maintenance. Consent from the patient or family to forgo (withhold or withdraw) quantitative futility may not be required, but qualitative futility requires at least assent prior to forgoing.

Clinicians' attitudes and values can affect the outcome of decisions about limits on interventions.[101] Decisions about medical futility are often based more on value judgments about whether a treatment is worth the subsequent amount of suffering and resources (financial and human) and its potential benefits and burdens than on any universally accepted definition of futility.[99] "Futility" is a term used by clinicians when they do not believe continuing the current level of care is "worth it." Futility is not a term used by patients or families. The use of value judgments is appropriate and necessary when making decisions about medical futility, but the judgments should be stated explicitly, not masked in language that implies standards of futility that do not exist.

In making a determination of qualitative futility, clinicians need to be mindful of the fact that this determination can be based on their own values and care preferences, and not necessarily on the values and care preferences of those for whom they are caring. Research has identified that the end-of-life care preferences of healthcare workers is relatively homogenous.[5,6] The end-of-life preferences of patients is more heterogeneous with some wanting to die without medical interventions (similarly to healthcare workers), but others wanting to "go out fighting."[9] When clinicians care for patients with values that are very different from their own, they sometimes develop hypotheses to explain why the family would want to keep the patient alive. These hypotheses may include that family members are benefitting monetarily by keeping the patient alive, that they do not understand the severity of the medical situation, or that they are unable to understand the situation because of cognitive impairments. When clinicians create these hypotheses, they may consciously or subconsciously interact in less respectful ways with family members. This, in turn, does not lead to an environment of trust or respectful disagreement. In one piece, Robert Truog writes about why performing futile CPR on a dying child was beneficial for the family.[84] Finally, it is important for clinicians to remember that even if a family is keeping a patient alive for monetary reasons, that money is usually being used to support the family, not for nefarious reasons. If these patients could be awakened, many of them might feel that it was acceptable for their lives to be prolonged in order for their families to continue to have adequate housing and food.

When requests for futile or potentially inappropriate treatments arise, it is important to continue open communication with patients and surrogates. Communication techniques and conducting goals of care discussions are covered in depth in *UNIPAC 5*. When receiving such requests, it is important to consider what factors may be driving patients or surrogates to continue to request this type of care. Occasionally, family members of patients continuing to receive potentially inappropriate treatments may want to prolong their loved one's life as they wait for a potential "miracle" or divine intervention. This particular situation can be very challenging for clinicians to negotiate. Delisser describes a practical approach to patients and families who are waiting for miracles that involves exploring with the patient or surrogate the meaning and significance of a miracle to them as a first step.[80] Delisser advocates for taking a calm, nonargumentative response to surrogate explanations, and negotiating patient-centered compromises, while conveying respect for the patient's spirituality, and recognizes the need to practice good medicine.[80]

Decisions about medical futility or potentially inappropriate treatments should be made after the clinician, the patient or surrogate, family members, and members of an interdisciplinary team have

- participated in a decision-making process
- achieved a common understanding of the patient's medical condition and prognosis
- articulated the patient's goals of treatment
- fully disclosed a treatment's likely benefits and burdens from the patient's perspective
- examined reasons why a treatment might be unwarranted
- clarified misconceptions and unrealistic expectations
- explicitly stated the values that are informing the decision.

When a patient or surrogate is adamant about obtaining treatments that are likely to result in heavy burdens and few benefits, a patient can be discharged or transferred to another institution as a last resort. Before this occurs, every effort should be made to find common ground with the patient and family and an ethics consult should be considered to try to identify areas of compromise. If a case requires transfer to another provider or institution, a referral to the institution's ethics committee and legal department should be considered.

The concept of futility has been controversial, and attempts to implement it to limit treatment despite the wishes of the patient's family have led to serious disagreements.[102] Texas has enacted legislation giving clinicians the authority, upon approval of a hospital ethics committee, to remove life-sustaining medical treatment without consent of the patient or family under circumstances deemed medically futile.[103] Treatment can be removed even if removal is contrary to a patient's wishes or the patient cannot directly express his or her preferences and removal can be contrary to instructions in the patient's advance directive or the decision of the patient's healthcare proxy.[104] Under the Texas statute, judicial review is limited and the hospital ethics committee decision essentially is the final decision.[104] The clinicians and ethics committee members who remove treatments pursuant to this legislation are given immunity from civil and criminal liability.[104] The Texas law remains very controversial.[105,106] One analysis found that patients in 61% of the cases in which the law was enacted were African American.[107] This questions social justice and whether the law is applied equally to all members of the population.

More recently, the concept of futility relevant to ICU settings in particular has evolved and is articulated in a practice guideline titled "Responding to Requests for Inappropriate Treatments in Intensive Care Units" led by the American Thoracic Society and cosponsored by multiple critical care societies. This position is applicable in cases where surrogates request that life-prolonging interventions be tried or continued despite a perceived lack of benefit among clinicians caring for the patient. Moreover, this framework appears to be applicable to patients receiving potentially inappropriate treatments regardless of hospital unit (ie, not necessarily within an ICU setting). It entails four main points and recommendations as outlined in the sidebar Responding to Request for Potentially Inappropriate Treatments in Intensive Care Units.[10]

Responding to Requests for Potentially Inappropriate Treatments in Intensive Care Units[10]

1. Institutions should implement strategies to prevent intractable treatment conflicts, including proactive communication and early involvement of expert consultants.

2. The term "potentially inappropriate" should be used, rather than futile, to describe treatments that have at least some chance of accomplishing the effect sought by the patient, but clinicians believe that competing ethical considerations justify not providing them. Clinicians should explain and advocate for the treatment plan they believe is appropriate. Conflicts regarding potentially inappropriate treatments that remain intractable despite intensive communication and negotiation should be managed by a fair process of conflict resolution; this process should include hospital review, attempts to find a willing provider at another institution, and opportunity for external review of decisions. When time pressures make it infeasible to complete all steps of the conflict resolution process and clinicians have a high degree of certainty that the requested treatment is outside accepted practice, they should seek procedural oversight to the extent allowed by the clinical situation and need not provide the requested treatment.

3. Use of the term "futile" should be restricted to the rare situations in which surrogates request interventions that simply cannot accomplish their intended physiologic goal. Clinicians should not provide futile interventions.

4. The medical profession should lead public engagement efforts and advocate for policies and legislation about when life-prolonging technologies should not be used.

Withholding and Withdrawing Life-Sustaining Treatment

End-of-life care often involves withholding or withdrawing potentially life-sustaining treatment. *Life-sustaining treatment* is treatment that may keep the patient alive for at least a limited period of time. Courts have emphasized patient autonomy, recognizing that under the common law and the US Constitution, any adult patient with mental capacity is free to reject any form of medical treatment, including life-sustaining treatment. Although making the decision to withhold a treatment may be psychologically easier than making a decision to withdraw it, the decisions are legally and ethically equivalent. The US Supreme Court also has recognized that the withdrawal of life-sustaining treatment is not equivalent to physician-assisted dying. In *Vacco v Quill* (discussed in the Landmark Cases chapter), it states

> ...[We] think the distinction between assisting suicide and withdrawing life-sustaining treatment, a distinction widely recognized and endorsed in the medical profession and in our legal traditions, is both important and logical; it is certainly rational...The distinction comports with fundamental legal principles of causation and intent. First, when a patient refuses life-sustaining medical treatment, he dies from an underlying fatal disease or pathology; but if a patient ingests lethal medication prescribed by a physician, he is killed by that medication...Furthermore, a physician who withdraws, or honors a patient's refusal to begin, life-sustaining medical treatment purposefully intends, or may so intend, only to respect his patient's wishes and "to cease doing useless and futile or degrading things to the patient when [the patient] no longer stands to benefit from them." ...The same is true when a doctor provides aggressive palliative care; in some cases, painkilling drugs may hasten a patient's death, but the physician's purpose and intent is, or may be, only to ease his patient's pain. A doctor who assists a suicide, however, "must, necessarily and indubitably, intend primarily that the patient be made dead."...Similarly, a patient who commits suicide with a doctor's aid necessarily has the specific intent to end his or her own life, while a patient who refuses or discontinues treatment might not.[108]

The right to refuse life-sustaining medical treatment is not unlimited. It must balance the patient's autonomous right to bodily integrity against the state's interest in the preservation of life.[35] This state interest is, however, at its weakest when an adult patient with capacity who is terminally ill refuses life-sustaining treatment. The right to refuse life-sustaining treatment is virtually absolute when the decision is made by an adult patient with terminal illness with decision-making capacity. A patient is *terminally ill* when he or she will die in a relatively short period of time regardless of whether life-sustaining treatment is continued or withdrawn. The use of terminal illness as a "poor criterion" for determining whether treatment may be withheld[48] has been criticized, but withdrawing or withholding life-sustaining treatment at the request of a terminally ill patient with decision-making capacity involves no legal risk. Although patients can refuse all medical treatments, including those offered for palliation, offering palliative interventions for relieving physical, emotional, psychosocial, and spiritual pain is obligatory.

Although society and the legal system appear to have reached consensus that fully informed adult patients with capacity have the right to refuse all medical treatment including life-sustaining treatment without court intervention, even without the presence of terminal illness, the withdrawal of life-sustaining treatment from incapacitated patients is more problematic. In most states, judicial review is not routinely required to withhold or withdraw life-sustaining treatment from incapacitated patients.[35] Clinicians are ordinarily permitted to comply with the previous instructions given by a patient concerning withholding or withdrawing when the patient had decision-making capacity regardless of whether those instructions are contained in a formal legal document. In most states a properly designated surrogate may refuse life-sustaining treatment on behalf of an incapacitated patient without the necessity of judicial review of the decision.[35]

However, a particular barrier to withdrawing life-sustaining treatment occurs when a patient loses decisional capacity, does not have an advance directive and does not have involved family to act as surrogates. These patients are commonly assigned to a court-appointed guardian, who usually does not know the patient personally until the time he or she is assigned to the patient's case. Unfortunately, there is state variability regarding a court-appointed guardians' legal abilities to make end-of-life decisions and to withdraw life-sustaining treatments. In a number of states the laws governing the legal guardian's ability to make these decisions are complex, inconsistent, and incomplete.[109]

Although there is a widespread consensus that judicial review of a surrogate's decision is not routinely required to withdraw or withhold life-sustaining treatment from incapacitated patients, there may be cases in which some court involvement is appropriate or necessary under state law. There is higher risk for liability exposure when there is no advance directive to provide guidance and no prior surrogate appointment, especially if there is disagreement among family members or with the clinician regarding the appropriate course of treatment. Generally, clinicians and family members should meet and try to achieve consensus about what the patient would want under these circumstances. Palliative care and ethics consultation can help to seek consensus and resolve differences when possible.

Although there is no legal requirement that a clinician contact a hospital's legal counsel or risk management department before discontinuing life-sustaining treatment for incapacitated patients, policies at some hospitals may require this type of notification when clear consensus cannot be achieved due to legitimate concerns about liability under applicable state laws.

Decisions to withhold or withdraw life-sustaining treatment should be based on an analysis of the treatment's benefits and burdens relative to the patient's stated goals of care, prognosis, and determination of the quality of life that may result from the treatment.[110] The patient's wishes and medical indications should also be taken into consideration.

After a decision is made to withdraw a life-sustaining intervention, the primary concern is to withdraw it in the most humane way possible to avoid furthering the patient and family's suffering, prolonging the dying process, and using unnecessary resources.[111]

Guidelines for Withholding and Withdrawing Life-Sustaining Treatment

Although making the decision to forgo a treatment may be psychologically easier than making a decision to withdraw it, the decisions are usually ethically and legally equivalent.[112,113] A decision to withhold a feeding tube can be an ethical choice and so can a decision to remove the tube when the treatment's burdens exceed its benefits or when it no longer serves the goals of care. Initiating a treatment does not mandate its continued use until the patient dies.

Life-sustaining treatments are ethically neutral in themselves; their benefits and burdens cannot be determined apart from a specific patient's diagnosis and prognosis, beliefs and values, quality of life, goals of care, and medical indications for treatment.

When decisions must be made about withholding or withdrawing a life-sustaining treatment, the outcome of the decision-making process will differ depending on the treatment's benefits and burdens for a specific patient. For example, decisions about orthopedic surgery for a fracture are likely to differ when one patient is an otherwise healthy victim of an automobile accident and the other is a terminally ill patient with cancer, a pathological bone fracture, and a life expectancy of 2 days. Likewise, a child dying of leukemia with dyspnea from anemia could be treated with a blood transfusion, but forcing a blood transfusion on the dying child of a Jehovah's Witness family is likely to cause more harm than good regardless of the child's respiratory rate.

In most acute care situations, there is a "best" medical treatment, or one that restores patients to health most efficiently. In end-of-life care settings, in which returning patients to health is not an option, a treatment's likely effect on the quality (and length) of the patient's remaining life must be carefully considered. The mere availability of a medical treatment does not mandate its use. The existence of treatments such as artificial nutrition and hydration (ANH), ventilation, CPR, antibiotics, and dialysis does not mandate their use for every patient in every situation. Each treatment must be evaluated within the context of the patient's condition, values, and goals.

When the benefits of a palliative treatment are uncertain, offering a short trial of the treatment and then withdrawing it if it proves to be ineffective or burdensome may be preferable to not offering the treatment at all. Fears about withdrawal should not prohibit time-limited trials of disease-directed or palliative treatments that might benefit a patient.[114] For example, starting hydration intravenously or subcutaneously to treat a patient's delirium and then withdrawing it if it proves ineffective or causes pulmonary congestion may be preferable to withholding a potentially helpful intervention. When deciding to pursue a time-limited trial, the clinicians, patient, and family together should determine the length of the trial and identify clear, measurable, desired outcomes for the trial. Deciding to determine if the patient is "better" in 2 weeks may be difficult to assess. For example, a family may feel that a patient is "better" because his eyes are open more, but the clinicians may believe that the patient's overall condition has not changed.

Withdrawing unwanted and burdensome treatment is consistent with the ethical practice of medicine. When unwanted treatment is withdrawn and a patient subsequently dies from an underlying disease or condition, clinicians involved with the case are not morally culpable, nor have they caused the patient's death. Rather, by withdrawing unwanted life-sustaining treatments, clinicians have allowed the patient to die from the underlying illness or condition rather than artificially prolonging the dying process.[115] As technological capabilities increase, it is becoming less clear that patients die from a natural progression of their underlying disease when certain technologies are withdrawn such as left ventricular assist devices or cardiac pacemakers. However, most clinicians and ethicists believe these interventions can be stopped in the appropriate context.[116,117]

Ethically, clinicians are not required to prolong life against a patient's wishes. They should consider the benefits and burdens of treatments and the quality of any prolonged life that might result, but ultimately it is the patient's view of these considerations that overrides those of the clinicians. Rescuing a terminally ill patient from a potentially lethal complication may add a few days of life, but it also means the patient may die of a future complication that might be more difficult to palliate.

Although most people believe life is good, few believe it should absolutely be protected or continued without regard to cost or circumstance. Some religious traditions place a high value on preserving life and demand the continuation of all possible measures designed to prolong life. In such cases, involving the patient's family members and religious advisers in discussions of proposed treatments can clarify issues and help resolve conflicts. In rare situations, conflict may continue until the patient dies; nevertheless, suffering usually can be alleviated even in these difficult situations.

Communication About Withholding and Withdrawing Treatment

Good communication with patients or surrogates about withholding or withdrawing treatment is essential. Patients may be more willing to experiment with treatments that might prove beneficial if they believe their wishes about withdrawal will be respected. Conversely, patients and family members often are more willing to withdraw ineffective or burdensome treatments when they have been included in the decision-making process and understand the implications of continued treatment. In most cases, patients and families are willing to forgo life-sustaining treatments that offer little hope of benefit.[118]

When communicating with patients or surrogates and families about treatments, clinicians should discuss the potential benefits and burdens of specific treatments for the patient as well as advise on the issue of time-limited trials, if applicable. Clinicians also should discuss withdrawing treatments when they become ineffective or when their burdens outweigh their benefits. Clinicians also must be aware of potential conflicts that might arise regarding the patient's or surrogate's cultural and religious beliefs and values. Culturally competent health care in an increasingly diverse population requires awareness of the importance of culture, particularly spirituality and religion and race and ethnicity, in the care of hospitalized patients at the end of life.[119-122] When it is unclear whether culture or religion may be factoring into a decision, clinicians can demonstrate cultural humility, asking open-ended questions to better understand their patient's perspective.[123]

AAHPM Position Statement on Withholding and Withdrawing Nonbeneficial Medical Interventions[124]

Approved by the AAHPM Board of Directors November 2011

Background

Palliative care seeks to relieve suffering associated with life-limiting illness. As illness progresses, there may also be times when the burdens of medical interventions outweigh their benefits, when the intervention is nonbeneficial, or when its use is inconsistent with the patient's goals. Consideration of withdrawing or withholding such interventions is then appropriate. Examples of specific interventions that may be withdrawn or withheld include, but are not limited to, ventilatory support, hemodialysis, implanted cardiac defibrillators (ICDs), cardiopulmonary resuscitation (CPR), vasopressors, artificial (assisted) nutrition/hydration, and antibiotics.

Statement

AAHPM endorses the ethically and legally accepted view that withholding and withdrawing nonbeneficial medical interventions are morally indistinguishable, and are appropriate when consistent with the patient's goals of care. Withdrawing or withholding nonbeneficial medical interventions is acceptable throughout the course of progressive, life-limiting illness, although patients with whom these discussions are held are often close to death.

When considering withholding or withdrawing a nonbeneficial medical intervention, clinicians should systematically:

- Assess the decision-making capacity of the patient. For patients lacking capacity, review all appropriate advance care planning documents and discuss decisions about withholding and withdrawing interventions with the designated surrogate decision maker, who should use substituted judgment. It is the responsibility of the physician and all members of the care team to keep the focus of decision making on the patient's preferences and best interests, rather than on the surrogate's beliefs.

- Identify the overall goals of treatment and care for the patient, considering the current disease status and the social, familial, psychological, and spiritual dimensions of the patient's situation.

- Identify the intended goals of the intervention under consideration, including the potential burdens and benefits of that therapy.

- Assess the burdens and benefits of starting (or withholding) or continuing (or withdrawing) an intervention. The assessment should include objective medical data, an assessment of the likely outcome for the patient with the proposed intervention, as well as alternative interventions. When the outcome of a proposed intervention is uncertain, clinicians should consider a time-limited trial of the specific intervention.

- Make a recommendation concerning continuing/starting or withdrawing/withholding a nonbeneficial intervention that is based on the patient's values, goals, and expected likelihood of success.

- Explain what treatments will be continued and what additional treatments will be added if a specific medical intervention is to be withheld or withdrawn and emphasize the types of support that can be provided to either the patient or family. Engage an ethics committee or other institutional committee in cases of disagreement.

Ethical Principles

Support for withholding or withdrawing nonbeneficial medical interventions is rooted in Western biomedical ethics and American law. The key ethical features including the following:

- A major goal of medicine is to relieve suffering.

- In the Western biomedical ethical tradition, there is no moral distinction between withdrawing and withholding a medical intervention. Clinicians should recognize, however, that there may be cultural, religious, or psychological reasons for patients and families to be concerned about withdrawing or withholding interventions. Clinicians should strive to understand the basis for the perspective of patients and families and to reconcile their views with standard practice when possible.

- Clinicians should respect patient autonomy, as directly expressed by the patient, or through a surrogate. However, clinicians should not implement therapies that cannot accomplish the patient's goals of care.

- Imbedded within patient autonomy or self-governance is the notion of patient rights. All should remember that the negative right to be left alone, to refuse an offered intervention, is stronger than a positive right to receive something demanded but not offered.

- The patient should give informed consent; if the patient lacks decision-making capacity, the surrogate decision maker should give informed consent consistent with the goals of care and the patient's values.

- Withholding or withdrawing of nonbeneficial interventions is ethically and legally distinct from physician-assisted suicide and euthanasia. Withholding or withdrawing of nonbeneficial interventions is ethically appropriate even if the death of a patient occurs closely following withdrawal of therapy.

Role of Artificial Nutrition and Hydration

Clinical Situation

Mrs. Steinbeck

Mrs. Steinbeck is a 94-year-old nursing home resident with advanced dementia, atrial fibrillation, osteoporosis, and osteoarthritis. Her grandson, Eli, lives a few hours away. She never completed an advance directive.

On her latest hospitalization, Mrs. Steinbeck was intubated for pneumonia but was able to be extubated after 3 days. Her code status was full code. She was nonverbal and easily agitated when turned, cleaned, or given nursing care. She was placed in four-point restraints after repeatedly striking out at anyone trying to provide care, and she was getting only occasional as-needed doses of haloperidol. A formal swallow evaluation confirmed that she was consistently aspirating, and the team had scheduled her for a percutaneous gastrostomy (PEG) tube insertion after a brief phone call to her grandson. An alarmed nurse asked the medical team for a palliative care consult to talk with the family about prognosis, goals of care, and symptom management.

The palliative care nurse suggested a family meeting by phone with the attending physician, Mrs. Steinbeck's nurse, the case manager on the floor, and other family members to discuss Mrs. Steinbeck's future and what other interventions might also be options. This meeting took place the next afternoon. During the family meeting, the attending physician reviewed her recent medical decline and confirmed that this would continue until death. Eli and his wife both said that they would not want to prolong her life, given her prognosis, especially because she seemed to have no awareness of her surroundings. Instead of the PEG, the family decided to change her code status to DNAR and, with the medical team, agreed to stop the warfarin because the risks, given her illness and lack of oral intake as well as the discomfort caused by blood draws, were felt to be greater than the low risk of a stroke from atrial fibrillation. The family and medical team agreed to transfer her back to her nursing home, where she was known and comfortable, and to have a contracted local hospice visit her there. Because nutrition was important to Eli and his wife, the hospice team subsequently recommended that the nursing home staff try hand feedings and thickened liquids.

Clinicians need to facilitate honest and thoughtful conversations with patients and their families about artificial nutrition and hydration (ANH), which also is referred to as medically assisted nutrition and hydration. ANH is a medical procedure that involves placing a tube or needle into the alimentary tract, into a vein, or under the skin to deliver fluids and nutrients. It does not refer to assisted oral feeding, such as putting a cup to the patient's mouth or spooning or syringing liquid into a patient's mouth. Expectations, relative benefits, limitations and potential long-term treatment burdens of ANH need to be thoughtfully considered and clarified

The literature suggests that the benefits from the use of ANH in many palliative care patients may be limited, yet the risks and treatment burdens of ANH are substantial. To address this topic, position statements have been released in recent years from several medical societies aimed at increasing awareness among providers and patient consumer groups[125] (see AAHPM position statement on ANH on page 46). Moreover, a pair of *Cochrane* reviews published in 2014 concluded there was insufficient evidence to make any recommendation regarding medically assisted nutrition or hydration in palliative care patients.[126,127]

Although there have been no randomized controlled studies examining the use of feeding tubes, as this type of study would be difficult to conduct, substantial observational studies exist that have captured relevant outcomes important for patients with advanced illness. For example, a large prospective study of patients with dementia residing in US nursing homes who had developed recent difficulties with eating showed that a feeding tube insertion did not result in a survival benefit.[128] This study confirmed the findings of a number of smaller, prior observational studies involving patients with dementia that suggest a lack of evidence of prolonged survival rates associated with use of ANH.[113,115,116,129-131]

Most of the data about the long-term treatment burdens associated with tube feeding are drawn from the fairly robust studies of patients with advanced dementia (AD). Many outcomes other than survival that affect quality of life are important to consider in patients with any life-limiting illness, including AD. For example, it has been shown that tube feedings likely increase the risk for aspiration in patients with AD.[115] Furthermore, despite patients receiving adequate calories from tube feedings administered in long-term care facilities, evidence suggests that these patients may experience continued weight loss and depletion of lean and fat body mass.[121] Similarly, no studies have provided evidence that ANH improves the healing rate of pressure ulcers or other infections.[115,116,129] In fact, among patients with AD, feeding tubes are not associated with improved pressure ulcer healing, and appear to be associated with an increased risk of developing new pressure ulcers.[132]

Patients with dementia may pull on their PEG tubes, leading inpatient or nursing home staff to use restraining devices, which can exacerbate delirium or agitation, and also can worsen pressure ulcers. Notably, feeding tube–related complications accounted for 47% of emergency room visits in one prospective study of nursing home patients with AD.[133] In light of limited benefits and considerable longer term burdens of ANH therapy, clinicians should explore alternatives to ANH that are consistent with comfort-focused care, such as a careful hand-feeding program.[115,130]

A landmark prospective study characterizing the natural history and trajectory of advanced dementia has yielded important results informing palliative care approaches for this population. This study, called the CASCADE (choices, attitudes, and strategies for care of advanced dementia at the end of life) study, followed older adults with advanced dementia in 22 nursing homes over 18 months and found that mortality among these nursing home residents with AD was 25% at 6 months and 55% at 18 months.[134] Importantly, almost 90% developed eating problems as part of the progression of AD.[134] Subsequently, a number of practice guidelines and position statements have been published, advocating for careful hand-feeding and the avoidance of feeding tubes in patients with AD.[125,135]

Evidence regarding ANH for patients with cancer is difficult to interpret given the heterogeneous nature of the cancer population, including cancer type and disease progression. A recent systematic review found a lack of high-quality studies to guide practice recommendations regarding medically assisted nutrition (or ANH) for patients receiving palliative care.[127] Nonetheless, these authors note the existence of a few uncontrolled prospective studies that suggest there may be a role for ANH in patients with a prognosis of more than weeks to months, but that the decision needs to be highly individualized, taking into account risks of enteral or parenteral nutrition and overall goals of care. Several smaller, observational studies suggest that a subset of patients receiving total parenteral nutrition (TPN) experience increased survival rates of at least 3 months.[124,136] In a Mayo Clinic study conducted over a 20-year period from 1979 to 1999 involving 52 patients with a variety of cancers (most with bowel obstruction or malabsorption receiving home TPN), 16 survived for 1 year or longer. The investigators were not able to identify predictors for long-term survival and instead concluded that use of TPN must be determined on a case-by-case basis.[136] In cases of ovarian cancer complicated by bowel obstruction, one small study[137] noted modest benefit (approximately 2 weeks of extended survival) and another study showed no benefit with use of TPN.[138] Conversely, meta-analysis shows that TPN for patients with cancer receiving chemotherapy is associated with decreased survival, decreased response to chemotherapy, and an increased rate of infection.[139] Importantly, significant potential adverse effects associated with TPN include infection, hepatic dysfunction, electrolyte abnormalities, and thrombosis. Quality of life and patient considerations include the need for frequent monitoring of electrolytes and cost.[140]

One example of a specific patient population in which longer term enteral or parenteral nutrition may be a consideration includes those deemed to have a higher functional status but with terminal cancer and associated GI obstruction; however, this is an area without a good evidence base and in need of further study.[141] Although it is generally accepted that ANH is not indicated to address an anorexia/cachexia syndrome, there may be a potential role for ANH in those patients with advanced illness who are unable to effectively swallow but have an otherwise potentially longer prognosis (ie, months to years) when considering the trajectory of their underlying condition (eg, motor neuron disease or head and neck cancer) than they would from an acute dysphagia or GI obstruction.[127] Although there are limited data regarding the overall utility of ANH in most patients at end of life, there are indications for this therapy in some patients with ALS, esophageal or other obstructive malignancies, or acute stroke syndromes.[142] Given the lack of strong evidence to guide these decisions, clinicians must carefully weigh patient preferences and goals of care along with known risks, longer term treatment burdens, and perceived benefits when proposing all forms of ANH and engaging patients in shared decision-making processes.[143]

Efforts to document improvements from parenteral hydration for patients with advanced cancer have not been successful.[122,126] Although no robust evidence base currently exists to support the role of hydration near the end of life, hydration may be a goal for some patients and clinicians in an attempt to address certain symptoms, despite known associated complications.[140] To meet the goal of hydration, a short-term trial of intravenous fluids or hypodermoclysis[144] may be worthwhile to help mitigate mental status changes, generalized weakness, or malaise in patients with an anticipated life expectancy of at least several days. Hypodermoclysis offers the advantage of avoiding the need to establish peripheral intravenous access.[145,146] A small study has shown that parenteral hydration may alleviate sedation and myoclonus (but not fatigue or hallucinations) for several days in patients who are dehydrated.[147] However, a more recent, larger, randomized study showed no difference among hospice patients with advanced cancer receiving hydration of 1 liter per day with regard to symptoms, quality of life, or survival compared with placebo.[148] Clinicians need to educate patients and families about the increased risk of third-space fluid retention and respiratory congestion with parenteral hydration or TPN, reinforcing the need to frequently reassess the benefits of therapy.[140]

Clinicians need to make sure that families understand a lack of nutrition and fluids does not appear to increase suffering for dying patients; in fact, decreased intake is a normal part of the dying process. Most clinicians and nurses who are familiar with end-of-life care will document that patients do not appear to experience hunger or thirst, do not request food or fluid beyond a taste or mouth moistening, and remain comfortable and peaceful as long as other symptoms are aggressively controlled.[147] Death most commonly occurs due to progression of the underlying illness, not a lack of food or fluids. Despite this, clinicians need to observe cultural and spiritual sensitivities that may influence a patient's or family's insistence on the continuation of ANH even when there may be little or no perceived medical benefit in continuing the intervention. The burdens and potential benefits should be thoroughly explored in these patients, with careful consideration of a patient's previously stated wishes and their prognosis. Opinions about the value of nutrition and hydration at the end of life vary widely.[149] The clinician should involve an interdisciplinary team, including a chaplain or other spiritual advisor appropriate for the patient, in periodic discussions about goals of care and whether ANH therapy continues to meet those goals.

Withdrawal of Artificial Nutrition and Hydration: Ethical Considerations

The goal of palliative care is to offer comfort and to support the development of care plans that are consistent with the patient's value system.[138] Clinicians should consider the withdrawal of ANH within an ethical framework, using all of the medical data available. As with other medical interventions, ANH should have a clearly defined therapeutic goal.

The decision to withdraw ANH is complicated by many issues. There is debate and uncertainty among the general public and some care providers about whether this is a basic need or a medical intervention. The fear of death by starvation and dehydration remains an emotionally charged subject. The public dialogue has focused mostly on ANH for younger patients in persistent vegetative states as opposed to adults dying of underlying terminal illnesses.[144,147,150] Withdrawal or withholding of ANH continues to be a particularly troublesome issue with respect to patients who are permanently unconscious or in a persistent vegetative state. When asked to rank their likelihood of withdrawing eight life-sustaining treatments, a group of 481 physicians indicated they would be least likely to withdraw tube feedings and intravenous fluids.[111]

Although consensus has apparently been reached about withdrawing ventilators from this group of patients, withdrawing ANH remains problematic for many family members and healthcare providers. With respect to patients dying of an underlying terminal illness, the withdrawal or withholding of ANH is a less contentious issue due to ANH possibly being medically inappropriate. Often, understanding the patient's or surrogate's spiritual and faith background can be helpful to guide decision making.

Catholic Healthcare Directives

The 2009 version of *Ethical and Religious Directives for Health Care Services,* 5th edition[142] (the norms adopted by Catholic bishops in the United States that apply to Catholic hospitals) states

56. A person has a moral obligation to use ordinary or proportionate means of preserving his or her life. Proportionate means are those that in the judgment of the patient offer a reasonable hope of benefit and do not entail an excessive burden or impose excessive expense on the family or the community.

57. A person may forgo extraordinary or disproportionate means of preserving life. Disproportionate means are those that in the patient's judgment do not offer a reasonable hope of benefit or entail an excessive burden, or impose excessive expense on the family or the community.

58. In principle, there is an obligation to provide patients with food and water, including medically assisted nutrition and hydration for those who cannot take food orally. This obligation extends to patients in chronic and presumably irreversible conditions (eg, the "persistent vegetative state") who can reasonably be expected to live indefinitely if given such care. Medically assisted nutrition and hydration become morally optional when they cannot reasonably be expected to prolong life or when they would be "excessively burdensome for the patient or [would] cause significant physical discomfort, for example resulting from complications in the use of the means employed." For instance, as a patient draws close to inevitable death from an underlying progressive and fatal condition, certain measures to provide nutrition and hydration may become

excessively burdensome and therefore not obligatory in light of their very limited ability to prolong life or provide comfort.

59. The free and informed judgment made by a competent adult patient concerning the use or withdrawal of life-sustaining procedures should always be respected and normally complied with, unless it is contrary to Catholic moral teaching.

A judicial consensus has emerged that ANH is medical treatment and may be refused under the same standards as other medical treatments, and there is now no question that adult patients with decision-making capacity can refuse ANH.[35] In the aftermath of the *Cruzan* case (see page 80), many states revised their advance directive and proxy appointment statutes to permit refusal of ANH.[35] But sometimes the instructions in an advance directive may not clearly address the situation.[149] Some states by statute limit the right of surrogates to refuse ANH.[35] In some states, withholding or withdrawing ANH from incapacitated patients who are not terminally ill may require court approval or other requirements such as proof of the patient's wishes by "clear and convincing" evidence.[37]

ANH may cause harm to dying patients. Large quantities of formula delivered by nasogastric or gastrostomy tubes can cause gastric distention, nausea, vomiting, diarrhea, dyspnea, and aspiration pneumonia.[151]

Despite evidence-based guidelines,[152] intravenous feedings can be associated with frequent venipuncture, the need for restraints to protect feeding lines, increased edema, ascites, pleural effusions, and pulmonary congestion. Patient selection for these therapies still is researched and debated.[141] Slowing the difficult process of dying sometimes is viewed as harmful by patients or their proxies.

If a medical treatment is causing harm or is not achieving its therapeutic goal, it should be withdrawn. The patient or surrogate and family should be included in this decision, provided with information regarding the reasons for discontinuing treatments, and informed of the interventions that will be used to keep the patient comfortable.

Patients or their surrogates may decide that a medical treatment such as ANH is too burdensome, even when a clinician or members of an interdisciplinary team believe it should be continued. Families may request ANH for their loved one who is losing weight. In such cases, the clinician should provide education about the treatment's potential benefits and burdens and investigate whether the treatment is for the patient's or family's benefit (eg, to help lessen family discomfort while watching a loved one get thinner or to address fears of "starving them to death"). A time-limited trial to determine the treatment's efficacy for the patient can be discussed. Distressing symptoms such as diarrhea, nausea, and edema caused by tube feedings can be relieved by decreasing the rate or concentration of the feedings, diluting the feedings with water, or adding metoclopramide to speed gastric emptying and reduce nausea. The treatment can be discontinued when the patient's condition or appropriate time-limited trials indicate that the therapeutic goal is not achievable, when the intervention has become more burdensome than beneficial, or when it no longer serves the patient's goals.[139] For example, if weight loss or overall decline occurs despite use of ANH, the clinician can recommend its cessation. Other agreed-upon complications, conditions, or recognition of lack of benefit may also lead to ANH discontinuation.[143]

AAHPM Statement on Artificial Nutrition and Hydration Near the End of Life[153]

Approved by the AAHPM Board of Directors September 13, 2013
(Replaces 2001 and 2006 Statements on Use of Nutrition and Hydration)

Background

Artificial nutrition and hydration (ANH) were originally developed to provide short-term support for patients who were acutely ill. For patients near the end of life, ANH is unlikely to prolong life and can potentially lead to medical complications and increase suffering. Researchers have found that ANH often leads to complications in patients nearing the end of life. Patients with advanced, life-limiting illness often lose the ability to eat and drink and/or interest in food and fluids. Ethical issues may arise when patients, families, or caregivers request ANH even if there is no prospect of recovery from the underlying illness or to accrue appreciable benefit.

Statement

AAHPM endorses the ethically and legally accepted view that ANH, whether delivered parenterally or through the gastrointestinal tract via a tube (including nasogastric tubes), is a medical intervention. Like other medical interventions, it should be evaluated by weighing its benefits and burdens in light of the patient's clinical circumstances and goals of care. ANH may offer benefits when administered in the setting of acute, reversible illness, or as a component of chronic disease management, when the patient can appreciate the benefits of the treatment and significant burdens are not disproportionate. Near the end of life, some widely assumed benefits of ANH, such as alleviation of thirst, may be achieved by less invasive measures including good mouth care or providing ice chips. The potential burdens of ANH depend on the route used and include sepsis (with total parenteral nutrition), aspiration, diarrhea (with tube feeding), pressure sores and skin breakdown, and complications due to fluid overload. In addition, agitated or confused patients receiving ANH may need to be physically restrained to prevent them from removing a gastrostomy tube, nasogastric tube, or central intravenous line.

AAHPM advocates respectful and informed discussions of the effects of ANH near the end of life among physicians, other healthcare professionals, patients, and families, preferably before the patient is close to death. It is incumbent on physicians, and other healthcare providers, to describe the options that exist when considering the implementation, continuation, or discontinuation of ANH, and establish goals of care with the patient and/or surrogate decision maker. Before the patient or family specify their preferences, the physician or other palliative care provider should ensure that they have adequate information to make a decision. The patient and family should also understand that appropriate medical interventions would continue, even if ANH is not implemented. Ideally, the patient will make his or her own decision about the use of ANH based on a careful assessment of potential benefits and burdens, consistent with legal and ethical norms that permit patients to accept or forgo specific medical interventions. Such choices are best made in concert with family, and should routinely be communicated to the patient's healthcare proxy. For patients who are unable to make or communicate decisions, the evaluation of benefits and burdens should be carried out by the patient's designated surrogate or next of kin, using substituted judgment whenever possible, in accordance with local laws.

AAHPM recognizes that in some faith traditions ANH is considered basic sustenance, and for some patients and families, ANH is of symbolic importance, apart from any measurable benefits for the patient's physical well-being. Such views should be explored, understood, and respected, in keeping with patient and family values, beliefs, and culture. Good communication is necessary to allow caregivers to learn about patient and family fears about "starvation" and other frequently expressed concerns. At the same time, communication is essential to explain the patient's clinical condition and that the inability to eat and drink can be a natural part of dying that is generally not associated with suffering. Judicious hand feeding and, in some situations, particularly if there is uncertainty about whether a patient will benefit from ANH, a time-limited trial of ANH may be useful. When a time-limited trial of ANH is pursued, clear, measurable end points should be determined at the beginning of the trial. The caregiving team should explain that, as with other medical therapies, ANH can be withdrawn if it is not achieving its desired purpose.

Key Elements

- Recognize that ANH is a form of medical therapy that, like other medical interventions, should be evaluated by weighing its benefits and burdens in light of the patient's goals of care and clinical circumstances.

- Acknowledge that ANH, like other medical interventions, can ethically be withheld or withdrawn, consistent with the patient's wishes and the clinical situation.

- Establish open communication between patients/families and caregivers, to assure that their concerns are heard and that the natural history of advanced disease is clarified.

- Respect patient's preferences for treatment, once the prognosis and anticipated trajectory with and without ANH have been explained.

Voluntary Stopping of Eating and Drinking

Although the concept of voluntary stopping of eating and drinking (VSED) is not new, it has gained national attention recently as a possible alternative to physician-assisted dying (PAD). To clarify, an accepted definition of VSED has been articulated as a "…conscious and deliberate decision, by a capacitated patient suffering from an advanced illness or an extremely debilitating medical condition, to intentionally refrain from receiving food or fluids by mouth, with the purpose of hastening death."[154]

VSED pertains to patients who retain full capacity to decide to voluntarily stop eating and drinking to have control over how and when they die. VSED usually pertains to someone who had been taking food and fluids orally until the point of VSED, and not to patients receiving ANH. It has been proposed that VSED be accepted as a potential "last resort" option for intractable terminal suffering, especially in states where PAD is not legal.[155] Despite the importance of the option of VSED to some patients, currently there exists a lack of evidence regarding qualitative patient symptoms and experiences, family perceptions, and provider experiences among those patients who have engaged in VSED.[156] Moreover, there have been no known observational studies conducted to assess the physiologic processes of patients undertaking VSED. More research is needed to formulate supportive practices and clinical guidelines for providers who are faced with patients attempting to pursue VSED.[156]

Quill proposes that VSED requests be evaluated the same as PAD requests, which includes a careful evaluation of the patient's intractable or unacceptable suffering, ensures access to high-quality palliative care, confirms the patient's full decision-making capacity, ensures a shared understanding of the patient's prognosis and medical condition, and, lastly, obtains a second opinion from another palliative care expert.[155] Furthermore, some patients strongly value their autonomy to the point of wanting to control how and when their death should take place. In states (or countries) where PAD is not legal, patients may opt for VSED as another palliative "last resort," although some of these patients may view this as an unnecessarily arduous path. Some patients may feel favorably about VSED, while still others may morally object to it.[155] Current literature and expert opinion suggests that all patients actively engaging in VSED continue to receive meticulous attention to symptom management through high-quality palliative care.[155,156]

A particularly challenging situation may arise when a patient loses capacity due to dementia or other forms of cognitive impairment. A competent patient has the right to refuse ANH and any other medical treatment, and can choose to engage in VSED. When a patient loses decisional capacity, decisions regarding ANH and any other medical treatment are addressed by the patient's proxy or surrogate decision maker in most cases. However, withholding food and fluids from a patient with dementia who appears to be readily accepting of food that is presented via careful handfeeding becomes problematic, especially in a nursing home setting where moral distress may ensue among staff providing care, and the nursing home is mandated to provide adequate food and water for patients.[157] For patients with advanced dementia, the notion of a "comfort feeding only" order is supported by palliative care expert opinion to allow for continuation of taste for pleasure while deemphasizing caloric intake and weights.[157,158] Menzel and Chandler-Cramer describe a compelling mechanism to incorporate the withholding of food and water by mouth through one's advance directive, to be triggered when one reaches a stage of dementia that meets predetermined criteria.[159] While this mechanism would allow for those who want to maintain their autonomy and control over how they die after they become incapacitated, multiple barriers currently exist within our healthcare system that would likely prevent a nursing home or other facility to legally implement and carry out such preferences as delineated in an advance directive. As the number of older adults with advanced dementia will continue to climb in the near future, the issue of withholding food and water from such a patient as indicated in an advance directive urgently needs further study for the medical community to consider acceptance of this practice.[157]

Palliative Sedation at the End of Life

Clinical Situation

Mr. Pratt

Mr. Pratt is a 72-year-old man with a history of radical surgery for prostate cancer that has metastasized to his pelvis and long bones. Mr. Pratt is referred for admission to a hospice inpatient unit because of a pain crisis. On admission, Mr. Pratt tells Dr. Cho that he "can't go on like this" and requests an injection of something to put him out of his misery. Mr. Pratt says he wouldn't allow an animal to suffer the way he is suffering and insists that he doesn't want to go on living. He says that he will ask his wife to buy a gun so he can shoot himself if the doctor won't help him die. Dr. Cho sits down to talk with Mr. Pratt.

During this conversation, Dr. Cho learns that Mr. Pratt has been prescribed long-acting morphine and ibuprofen. He has not taken the ibuprofen because of indigestion. The morphine dose managed his pain and allowed him to do things he enjoyed until a month ago, when his pain escalated. His oncologist suggested that he increase his morphine dose, but he felt too groggy on the increased dose. Mr. Pratt has been unable to sleep and feels hopeless, helpless, and worthless. Mr. Pratt wants to die because his pain is unbearable, and he no longer feels like a whole man because of his increasing dependence on his wife.

Dr. Cho reassures Mr. Pratt that there are interventions that may help his pain and that his outlook may improve if his pain is better controlled. Dr. Cho also mentions to Mr. Pratt that if these interventions are not successful at decreasing his pain, and if medication side effects are not acceptable, that another option exists, sedating him so he would no longer be aware of his pain. Mr. Pratt expresses relief to hear that there are still interventions available to reduce his pain, and that there are options besides hastening his death. He comments that he believes that ending his own life might conflict with his religious values, but he felt desperate.

According to the National Hospice and Palliative Care Organization (NHPCO), *palliative sedation* is the "lowering of patient consciousness using medications for the express purpose of limiting patient awareness of suffering that is intractable and intolerable."[160] Palliative sedation to relieve intractable and intolerable symptoms at the end of life is legal in the United States and is accepted as a reasonable treatment modality by 99% of AAHPM physicians surveyed.[161] Interdisciplinary palliative care teams use this strategy as a last resort to control symptoms by administering sedative medications in a controlled manner to intentionally reduce patient consciousness to the minimum extent necessary to render intolerable and refractory suffering tolerable.[160] Palliative sedation includes respite and continuous sedation. Respite sedation is sedation for a limited time with subsequent removal of sedation to reassess the patient. The NHPCO notes that for most patients, palliative sedation to less than total unconsciousness may allow the patient to rest comfortably but to still be aroused[160] (see **Table 7**).

A 2015 *Cochrane* review of palliative pharmacological sedation for terminally ill adults noted that currently, there is insufficient evidence that palliative sedation improves quality of life or symptom control.[163] Studies currently indicate that palliative sedation does not hasten death.[162-164] More high-quality research is needed to examine best practices and optimal outcomes of palliative sedation.[163]

A 2014 review examined nine palliative sedation guidelines from European, Canadian, Japanese, and American organizations.[165] The majority of these guidelines, as well as the views of American Medical Association and AAHPM, have agreed that patients being considered for palliative sedation must have a terminal illness in which death is imminent, and intractable distressing symptoms have been refractory to the most aggressive palliative care interventions. These symptoms include delirium, dyspnea, pain, nausea and vomiting, shortness of breath, uncontrolled bleeding, and myoclonus. Existential suffering remains a controversial indication for palliative sedation,[165] as it is unclear if existential suffering can be treated effectively with sleep or a reduced level of consciousness.[162] Another concern is that patients treated with palliative sedation may continue to suffer but are unable to communicate.[162]

Palliative sedation requires a physician with experience in palliative care to lead the intervention, and palliative care team members must have training and competence in palliative sedation.[160,165] The guidelines also state that palliative sedation must be carefully and explicitly explained to the patient or surrogate, and informed consent must be obtained.[165-167] The decision to pursue palliative sedation should be discussed with other healthcare professionals involved in the patient's care, as well. Likewise, gaining input from an ethics committee and conferring with other palliative medicine colleagues may also be helpful in complex cases involving refractory symptoms that may warrant palliative sedation. This type of collaboration may also mitigate the potential moral distress experienced by some providers.

Before instituting palliative sedation, the following conditions should be met[168]:

- A policy and procedure should be in place and followed.
- The patient is diagnosed with a terminal illness with a short prognosis.

- All palliative treatment has been exhausted and profound symptoms persist.
- A psychological assessment has been made.
- A spiritual assessment has been made.
- There is a DNAR order.
- There is informed consent.
- ANH was discussed before sedation.
    - » Appropriate documentation is ensured.
    - » Complicated grief bereavement follow-up for family is available.

Palliative sedation is achieved with benzodiazepines or barbiturates, which are usually administered intravenously or subcutaneously.[169] The dosage is rapidly titrated until signs

Table 7. Summary of Palliative Sedation

Definition	The lowering of patient consciousness using medications for the express purpose of limiting patient awareness of suffering that is intractable and intolerable
Appropriate patient population	Patients with terminal illness, with comfort focused goals, who are imminently dying
Widely accepted indications	Intractable distressing symptoms refractory to the most aggressive palliative care interventions. Symptoms include delirium, dyspnea, pain, nausea and vomiting, shortness of breath, urinary retention due to clot formation, gastrointestinal pain, uncontrolled bleeding and myoclonus.
	Palliative sedation for existential suffering remains controversial.
Key personnel	Physician with expertise in palliative care
	Interdisciplinary team, and patient/family must determine when symptoms are intolerable and intractable.
	All participating healthcare professionals should agree with the plan for sedation, or be given the option to opt out of the patient's care.
Consent	Informed consent from patient or surrogate
Other considerations	DNAR order in place
	Decisions regarding ANH made prior to discussion about palliative sedation
	Pain medications continued at current doses, since pain cannot be assessed once sedation has begun.

of discomfort have ceased. Patients are not necessarily sedated until they are unconscious. Opioids alone are not the medications of choice for inducing sedation; generally they are ineffective and induce unwanted side effects such as agitation and myoclonus. While sedated, patients should continue receiving medications such as opioids to relieve pain and other symptoms.[170,171] Updated guidelines exist on specific medications and dosages that can be used for palliative sedation in patients with refractory symptoms at the end of life.[172]

AAHPM Palliative Sedation Position Statement[167]

Approved by the AAHPM Board of Directors on December 5, 2014

Background

Palliative care supports patients whose diseases are associated with significant burden. Distressing symptoms exist on a spectrum from the most easily treated to the most refractory. Although preservation of awareness at the end of life is viewed as a priority for many, for some, the relief of symptoms may outweigh the desire to be conscious. Palliative sedation, as defined in this statement, is the intentional lowering of awareness towards, and including, unconsciousness for patients with severe and refractory symptoms.

Statement

A primary objective of palliative medicine is the easing of suffering via pharmacologic and nonpharmacologic techniques. As with any medical procedure, palliative sedation must satisfy the criteria of having a specific clinical indication, a target outcome, and a benefit/risk ratio that is acceptable to both the clinician and patient. Palliative sedation is an intervention reserved for extreme situations. The use of palliative sedation should only be considered after all available expertise to manage the target symptom has been accessed. The level of sedation should be proportionate to the patient's level of distress. As with all treatments, patients, when able, should participate in the decision to use palliative sedation. Treatment of other symptoms should be continued alongside palliative sedation, because sedation may decrease the patient's ability to communicate or display discomfort.

Palliative sedation raises ethical concerns when it significantly reduces patient consciousness to the degree that the patient is unable to substantially interact with others, does not have the ability or opportunity to change his mind, and is unable to eat and drink (thus potentially shortening survival in particular circumstances). Palliative sedation is ethically defensible when used 1) after careful interdisciplinary evaluation and treatment of the patient, 2) when palliative treatments that are not intended to affect consciousness have failed or, in the judgment of the clinician, are very likely to fail, 3) where its use is not expected to shorten the patient's time to death, and 4) only for the actual or expected duration of symptoms. Palliative sedation should not be considered irreversible in all circumstances. It may be appropriate, in some clinical situations when symptoms are deemed temporary, to decrease sedation after a predetermined time to assess efficacy, continued symptoms, and need for ongoing sedation.

In clinical practice, palliative sedation usually does not alter the timing or mechanism of a patient's death, as refractory symptoms are most often associated with very advanced terminal illness. Practitioners who use palliative sedation should be clear in their intent to palliate symptoms and to not shorten survival. Because patients receiving palliative sedation are typically close to death, most patients will no longer have desire to eat or drink. Artificial nutrition and hydration are not generally expected to benefit the patient receiving palliative sedation; however, questions about the use of artificial nutrition and hydration should be addressed before palliative sedation is undertaken. (See AAHPM position statement on page 46).

There is no clear consensus or scientific evidence regarding the most appropriate medication(s) to effect palliative sedation. As elsewhere in medicine, the agent should be selected based on safety, efficacy, and availability.

Although the Academy recognizes that existential distress may cause patients to experience suffering of significant magnitude, there is no consensus around the ability to define, assess, and gauge existential suffering, to measure the efficacy of treatments for existential distress, and whether it is in the realm of medicine to palliate such suffering when it occurs absent of physical symptoms. Patients with existential suffering should be thoroughly assessed and treated through vigorous multidisciplinary efforts which may include involving professionals who are not usual members of the palliative care team (eg, experts in psychology, family therapy, or specific spiritual services). If palliative sedation is used for truly refractory existential suffering, as for its use for physical symptoms, it should not shorten survival.

Physician-Assisted Dying

AAHPM defines *physician-assisted dying (PAD)* as "a physician providing, at the patient's request, a lethal dose of medication that the patient can take by his own hand to end otherwise intolerable suffering" (see AAHPM position statement on page 61). PAD, which also is referred to as physician-assisted suicide and also known as physician aid in dying, is distinguished from euthanasia, which refers to the act of directly ending another person's life by, for example, the administration of a lethal injection by the physician. Various terms have been used to describe actions taken by physicians on behalf of patients at the end of life (see **Table 8**).

Arguments For and Against Physician-Assisted Dying

With a few exceptions, consensus exists regarding the ethical appropriateness of withholding or withdrawing life-sustaining treatments at the request of a patient or surrogate (see Withholding and Withdrawing Life-Sustaining Treatment on page 34). In contrast, debate persists regarding the moral and ethical appropriateness of PAD and euthanasia.[173-175]

Table 8. Terminology Applied to Actions by Healthcare Providers in Dying Patients

Term	Alternate Terms	Illustrative Example
Legally permissible practices generally considered medical standard of care		
Withholding/withdrawing life-sustaining treatment	Allowing to die	Discontinuing ventilator support; forgoing artificial nutrition and hydration
Palliative sedation	Terminal sedation	Administering enough sedating medication to relieve refractory symptoms, with or without inducing unconsciousness
Double effect	"Risky dosing"; unintentional but potential hastening* of death by active symptom control in patient near death	Intentionally providing adequate dose of medication to relieve symptoms despite risk of worsening patient's hypotension or respiratory depression (eg, during terminal ventilator withdrawal)
Controversial practices legally permissible in some states but with evolving legal standards		
Physician-assisted death**	Aid in dying, "death with dignity," physician-assisted suicide	Providing patient with a prescription of lethal dose of medication for self-administration
Controversial practices generally not legally permissible but with evolving legal standards		
Voluntary euthanasia†	Voluntary active euthanasia; "mercy killing"	Administering lethal dose of medication at a person's request
Involuntary euthanasia†	"mercy killing"	Administering lethal dose of medication without a person's request, such as a person who is unconscious or lacks capacity to make such a request

*"Hastening of death" is theoretical, since it is not possible to pinpoint precise time of death.
**Legal in certain states only
†Not legal in any US state, but legal is some other countries.

The following arguments have been raised in opposition to PAD:

- Nonmaleficence. Physicians are obliged to "do no harm" to a patient and therefore have a professional obligation to not participate in assisted death. Furthermore, professional codes of ethics do not support PAD.[166,176-178]
- Patient autonomy is not unlimited and must give way to universal moral principles, such as the sanctity of human life and the avoidance of killing.
- Religious proscriptions. Under most religious traditions, intentionally ending another person's life, even at that person's request, is wrong.[179]
- Palliative care. Pain and suffering can be alleviated with skillful palliative interventions, including palliative (terminal) sedation. Requests for assisted death may be withdrawn when pain and depression are effectively addressed.
- Risks to society. Social policies that condone killing pose risks of a slippery slope that would lead to elimination of vulnerable groups such as disabled, elderly, or patients posing a financial burden on families or the healthcare system.
- Vulnerable groups. While opinions about PAD are mixed, even among vulnerable groups, some vulnerable populations are less likely than others to support this practice.[180]
- Societal trust of the health professions. This will deteriorate if medicine becomes an instrument of death.
- Financial motivation. By providing a less costly alternative to life-sustaining treatments, the practice of PAD might take precedence over "interventions that might otherwise enhance the quality of life for patients who are dying."[181]

The following arguments have been raised in favor of PAD:

- Beneficence and compassion. The physician has the duty to ease the suffering resulting from uncontrollable physical, emotional, or existential pain and should be able to provide the means for such a person to end his or her life.
- Patient autonomy. A patient whose disease causes unremitting suffering should be permitted to determine at what stage of the disease and the manner in which life may end. Refusal to participate in assisted death violates the principle of autonomy.
- Availability of safeguards. It is possible to formulate and implement guidelines to protect vulnerable persons from PAD to which they might be unwilling or unable to consent.
- Many patients who have been given medication to end their life do not ultimately use it for that purpose.[182] In such cases, having access to the medication can benefit the patient by providing reassurance that help will be available if necessary.

The "rightness" or "wrongness" of PAD will continue to be debated. Opinion surveys are not definitive, even if such methods were known to be perfectly reliable. Opinion polls of clinicians and the public over the last several decades have shown considerable variability, depending on the population studied, geographic area, year when data were obtained, method used, and the current high-profile events communicated in the media. Legislative initiatives have both supported and failed to support PAD, and public referenda likewise have both succeeded and failed. Finally, as noted earlier, professional medical associations have generally been opposed to PAD, but not invariably,[183] with some taking a neutral stance.[184,185] It remains to be seen how opinions and positions will evolve in the future.

Physician-Assisted Dying and the Law

Given an increasingly pluralistic society, along with rapid changes in medical technology and institutional structures, it is likely that ethical and moral debates will continue. Nonetheless, changes in the ethical and legal climate in the United States have taken place since the late 1960s, which saw the growth of the consumer-driven "right to die" movement, and the birth of the statutory living will in 1976.[186] During the two decades that followed, all states passed advance directive laws and many appellate courts affirmed the right of patients or their surrogate decision makers to refuse life-sustaining treatments. PAD, however, remained illegal in virtually all states, until two cases arguing for the right to PAD reached the US Supreme Court. In 1997, the Court rejected arguments that there is a constitutional right to PAD, finding that the statutes forbidding PAD in the states of Washington and New York did not violate the Constitution[108,187] (see Landmark Court Cases on page 73).

At the same time, however, the Supreme Court did not find that the Constitution explicitly forbids PAD. Thus, the Court's ruling, neither asserting a right to PAD nor prohibiting a state from legalizing it, left that particular power to the states, and much legal activity followed. Since the 1997 decisions, several states have legalized PAD by statute or appellate state court decision,[188,189] and legislation and legal appeals are pending in others. Shortly after Oregon passed the first statute legalizing PAD, the US Attorney General issued an interpretive rule that "prescribing, dispensing, or administering federally controlled substances" to cause death was not a legitimate medical purpose within the meaning of the Controlled Substances Act; therefore, a physician who did so would violate that act and risk revocation of his or her registration to dispense controlled substances.[190] This attempt was rebuffed by the US Supreme Court, which found that the Attorney General was not authorized to illegitimize a medical standard authorized under state law.[191] However, restrictions remain on the use of federal funds for PAD under federal statute,[192] which would affect, among other things, Medicare reimbursement, veterans' benefits, and federal employee participation in PAD. States that have legalized PAD are, nonetheless, in a position to provide guidance regarding alternative methods of payment for PAD.[193] Likewise, a federally employed clinician is not prohibited in any way from discussing end-of-life preferences with their patients. Guidance for responding to patients who request PAD has been published.[175,194,195]

Still, as of this writing, PAD is illegal in the majority of states. In fact, following the holdings in *Glucksberg* and *Vacco*, certain states created bans on assisted suicide or explicitly banned PAD by strengthening their existing criminal codes. No state has legalized the practice of euthanasia. Outside of the United States, PAD, including euthanasia, has been legalized in only a few countries. Certain features of laws in other countries are noted in the section titled Remaining Questions and Controversies (page 58) and are reviewed in detail in the References.[196,197]

State statutes that permit PAD in the United States generally* include the following requirements for the protection of patients:

- The patient is at least 18 years of age and is a resident of the state.
- The patient has a terminal illness or condition, defined as "an incurable and irreversible disease that has been medically confirmed and will, within reasonable medical judgment, produce death within 6 months."
- Clinical confirmation by a second physician of the patient's capacity and terminal condition; consultation by a mental health professional if mental illness exists that might impair the patient's judgment.
- Informed consent and witnessed decision by the patient; witnesses cannot be a close relative, someone entitled to a share of the estate, the attending physician, or staff of the facility where the patient is situated.
- A waiting period prior to receiving a prescription, to ascertain that the patient's decision is firm.
- "Lethal injection, mercy killing, or active euthanasia" are explicitly excluded as methods for aid-in-dying under the law.
- In addition, the laws include an opt-out clause providing immunity from any disciplinary action or sanction for a physician or other health professional who refuses to participate on the basis of a conscientious objection to PAD.

Why Do Patients Request Physician-Assisted Death?

Patient motivations for PAD are diverse. It has long been reported that requests are not necessarily due solely to pain or other physical symptoms.[201,202] Other patient concerns that are commonly voiced include inability to engage in activities that are important, enjoyable, or meaningful; loss of autonomy and being dependent on others; loss of control over the situation; loss of dignity; loss of control of bodily functions; being tired of life; and being a burden—financial or otherwise—to family, friends, or other caregivers.[201-204] Of note, evidence suggests that it is the fear of future pain, loss of control, or another potentially unendurable situation that could occur that leads to a request for PAD in advance of its actual occurrence.[204] In states where the practice is legal and follow-up information is available, between approximately 12% and 29% of people receiving prescriptions did not take the medication and died of other causes, according to recent data.[182,205] It is not known if failure to take the medications was due to imminent death from disease, a specific decision to forgo the medication, inability to ingest the medication, or other factors.

---

*These stipulations are generally common to existing statutes as of this writing. For details of specific provisions, see text of statutes.[190,198-200] It remains to be seen what methods will be used to regulate the practice in states that legalize PAD through high court decisions.

Some patients will bring up the topic of PAD with their physicians to begin a conversation about the end of life. These patients may not be clearly invested in pursuing this route. Physicians can use this opportunity to explore the patient's concerns about the end of life, even if they cannot prescribe the lethal medications. Limiting discussions to a statement that the physician does not participate can shut down future conversations about end-of-life treatment options.

Remaining Questions and Controversies

To date, no efforts exist in the United States to broaden the availability of PAD beyond strict criteria adopted by certain states; for example, a patient must be "terminally ill." Some conditions that do not satisfy the time-limited diagnosis may be particularly resistant to palliative care interventions, such as intractable depression, progressive neurological disease, fixed neurological deficits, and others. Commentators have supported or alluded to PAD in such circumstances, when patient suffering is extreme and the patient requests assistance in dying.[206-208] Such patients are sometimes able to receive PAD in certain other countries.[197,209,210]

Controversy particularly exists in situations when the disease itself creates incapacity, such as dementia. In such cases, assistance in dying would inherently be nonvoluntary. In one argument, PAD would be permissible for dementia, but only if the patient still retained capacity.[207] In a contrasting opinion, PAD could be practiced at a later stage, after loss of capacity, and ethical standards, including but not limited to advance directives, could be established that would justify this and prevent abuse.[211] At some point, however, the patient would be unable to undergo the process alone and would require more than a prescription, perhaps euthanasia. Currently, no state in the United State permits euthanasia in any situation.

PAD has been undertaken for psychiatric illness in Belgium[210] and the Netherlands,[212] reportedly in conjunction with established "due care criteria." The practice is permitted even in the absence of accompanying somatic illness and is not limited to severe depression but may occur in other psychiatric conditions when accompanied by intolerable suffering. In these circumstances, however, the patient's decisional capacity must be confirmed. Overall, much controversy remains regarding PAD in the context of psychiatric illness in North America and elsewhere.[213]

Perhaps most controversial is the practice of PAD in children, which is permitted in some countries in certain circumstances, such as emancipated minors. Recent law in Belgium also permits the practice for preadolescents if parents are in agreement, the child's death is expected in a short period of time, and an evaluation ascertains the child has the "capacity for discernment."[214] In the Netherlands, euthanasia is practiced in the case of severely impaired newborns, though perhaps uncommonly. This practice was not specifically legalized in the Dutch 2002 Euthanasia Act, which governed patients as young as 12 years of age. That law followed years of existing practice that was legally tolerated if a physician complied with standards set out years before,[201] and likely included some cases of euthanasia in the very young.[215,216]

After much debate regarding end-of-life decisions for newborns, strict, narrowly defined guidelines were promulgated by the Dutch Medical Association, which addressed the severely impaired newborn whose hopeless, fixed condition could not be addressed by palliative care or terminal withdrawal of life support. Criteria included, among others, parental consent, certainty of diagnosis and prognosis, and hopeless, unbearable suffering.[217,218]

AAHPM Advisory Brief: Guidance on Responding to Requests for Physician-Assisted Dying[219]

Background

Suffering near the end of life arises from many sources, including loss of sense of self, loss of control, fear of the future, and/or fear of being a burden upon others, as well as refractory physical and nonphysical symptoms. Rarely, patients seek the assistance of a physician to end their life. Physician-Assisted Dying (PAD) is defined as a physician providing, at the patient's request, a prescription for a lethal dose of medication that the patient can self-administer by ingestion, with the explicit intention of ending life. Although PAD has historically not been within the domain of standard medical practice, in recent years it has emerged as both an explicit and covert practice across various legal jurisdictions in the United States. PAD has become a legally sanctioned activity, subject to safeguards, first in Oregon in 1997 and, subsequently, in other states including Washington, Vermont, and California. As of the writing of this document, approximately one-sixth of the US population resides in a jurisdiction where PAD is legally permitted, and its legal status continues to evolve at the state level.

Purpose

The emphasis of this guidance statement is to entreat those medical providers who care for patients with terminal disease to understand the complexity of the request for assisted death, to provide an educated systematic response, and to use the best practices of palliative care to alleviate the suffering of patients that triggers a desire to pursue PAD. A primary goal of the American Academy of Hospice and Palliative Medicine (AAHPM) is to promote the development, use, and availability of palliative care to relieve patient suffering and to enhance quality of life while upholding respect for patients' and families' values and goals. The ending of suffering by ending life has been held as distinct from palliative care, which relieves suffering without intentionally hastening death.

AAHPM has a separate position statement on PAD that addresses ethical and social policy concerns.

Systematic Approach to Evaluate PAD Requests

Determine the nature of the request.

Is the patient seeking immediate assistance or considering the possibility of hastened death in the future? Is the patient airing thoughts about ending life without a specific intent or plan? Is the patient frustrated with living with illness, but not seriously contemplating ending life?

Clarify the cause(s) of intractable suffering.

Is there a loss of functional autonomy? Does the patient feel he or she is a burden or exhausted from prolonged dying? Is there severe pain or other unrelieved physical symptoms? Is the distress mainly emotional or spiritual?

Evaluate the patient's decision-making capacity.

Is there impairment affecting comprehension and judgment? Does the patient's request seem rational and proportionate to the clinical situation? Is the patient's request consistent with long standing values?

Explore emotional factors.

Do feelings of depression, worthlessness, excessive guilt, or fear substantially interfere with the patient's judgment? Does the patient have untreated or undertreated depression or other mental illness?

Explore situational factors.

Does the patient have a poor social network? Are there coercive influences such as looming bankruptcy? Is the patient subject to emotional, financial, or other forms of exploitation or abuse?

Initial Responses to PAD Requests.

- Utilize open-ended questions to understand the concerns that led the patient to request PAD.
- Respond empathically and strengthen the therapeutic relationship through respectful and nonjudgmental dialogue.
- Reevaluate and modify treatment of pain and all physical symptoms.
- Identify and address depression, anxiety, and/or spiritual suffering.
- Consult with experts in spiritual or psychological suffering when appropriate.
- Consult with colleagues experienced in palliative care/hospice as needed.
- Commit to the patient the intention of working toward a mutually acceptable solution for the patient's suffering.

When unacceptable suffering persists over a timeline often determined by the patient and the clinical course, despite systematic evaluation and standard palliative care intervention as outlined above, search for a mutually acceptable plan is essential. In these situations, consider the benefits and burdens of other alternatives including:

- discontinuation of potentially life-prolonging treatments such as steroids, insulin, oxygen supplementation, dialysis, or medically assisted hydration and nutrition
- voluntary cessation of oral intake if ethically acceptable to the patient and treating practitioners
- palliative sedation, potentially to unconsciousness, if suffering is intractable and severe.

Cautions

Despite consideration of this stepwise response, some patients will persist in a specific request for PAD. AAHPM advises great caution before pursuing PAD where legal, ensuring that

- the patient continues to receive the best possible palliative care coordinated with an interdisciplinary team and other nonpalliative care providers, irrespective of a decision to use PAD
- the patient has decisional capacity commensurate to the request for PAD
- the request is voluntary and not influenced by subtle or explicit coercion from any source
- all reasonable alternatives to PAD acceptable to the patient have been considered
- if the physician responds affirmatively to the request, he engages best available practices that limit avoidable suffering through end of life
- if the request conflicts with the physician's values, his response should take into account professional obligations of nonabandonment as well as the patient's ongoing clinical needs.

AAHPM Statement on Physician-Assisted Dying[220]

Approved by the AAHPM Board of Directors on June 24, 2016

Background

Suffering near the end of life arises from many sources, including loss of sense of self, loss of control, fear of the future, and/or fear of being a burden upon others, as well as refractory physical and nonphysical symptoms. Excellent medical care, including state-of-the-art palliative care, can address and help alleviate many sources of suffering. On occasion, however, patients seek the assistance of a physician to end their life.

Physician-Assisted Dying (PAD) is defined as a physician providing, at the patient's request, a prescription for a lethal dose of medication that the patient can self-administer by ingestion, with the explicit intention of ending life. Although PAD historically has not been within the domain of standard medical practice, in recent years it has emerged as both an explicit and covert practice across various legal jurisdictions in the United States. PAD has become a legally sanctioned activity, subject to safeguards, first in Oregon in 1997 and, subsequently, in other states including Washington, Vermont, and California. As of the writing of this document, approximately one-sixth of the US population resides in a jurisdiction where PAD is legally permitted, and its legal status continues to evolve at the state level.

A primary goal of the American Academy of Hospice and Palliative Medicine (AAHPM) is to promote the development, use, and availability of palliative care, including hospice, to relieve patient suffering and to enhance quality of life while upholding respect for patients' and families' values and goals. The ending of suffering by ending life has been held as distinct from palliative care, which relieves suffering without intentionally hastening death.

Statement

Situations in which Physician-Assisted Dying (PAD) is requested are challenging for physicians and other healthcare practitioners because they raise significant clinical, ethical, and legal issues. A diversity of positions exists in society, in medicine, and among members of the American Academy of Hospice and Palliative Medicine (AAHPM). AAHPM acknowledges that morally conscientious individuals adhere to a broad range of positions on this issue.

AAHPM takes a position of studied neutrality on the subject of whether PAD should be legally permitted or prohibited. However, as a matter of social policy, the Academy has concerns about a shift to include PAD in routine medical practice, including palliative care. Such a change risks unintended long-range consequences that may not yet be discernable, including effects on the relationship between medicine and society, the patient and physician, and the perceived or actual integrity of the medical profession. Any statutes legalizing PAD and related regulations must include safeguards to appropriately address these concerns, such as limiting eligibility to individuals with decision-making capacity with a limited life expectancy.

Social policy concerns notwithstanding, the Academy recognizes that in particular circumstances some physicians assist patients in ending their lives. Efforts to augment patients' psychosocial and spiritual resources so that they are better able to manage their suffering may make palliative treatments of physical symptoms more effective and may make these circumstances rarer. Nevertheless, some patients will continue to desire PAD.

Physicians practicing in jurisdictions in which PAD is legally permitted should never be obligated to participate in PAD if they hold moral or professional objections, nor should they be prohibited from participating within parameters defined by relevant statutes and terms of employment. Physicians who affirmatively respond to requests for PAD are obligated to ensure their actions are consistent with best available practices that limit avoidable suffering through end of life.

When a request for PAD is made by a terminally ill patient, medical practitioners should carefully evaluate the patient's concerns precipitating the inquiry and address the sources. Requests originating from family should not be pursued without direct discussion with the patient. Requests for PAD from surrogates of incapacitated patients should not be considered due to the complexities of the ethics of surrogate decision-making. However, surrogates' concerns prompting the request should be fully explored.

Organ Donation

Organ procurement and transplantation is a potential source for concern, comfort, or both for palliative care patients and their families.[221] It is important to realize that organ donation without palliative care increases the risk of inadequate end-of-life care and complicated bereavement in the donor's family.[222-224] The Hospice and Palliative Nurses Association has a position statement titled, "The Role of Palliative Care in Organ and Tissue Donation."[225] Most patients are potential donors at the end of life. Absolute contraindications to organ donation are Creutzfeldt-Jakob disease and other neurodegenerative diseases associated with infectious agents and human immunodeficiency disease but not HIV infection alone.[222] Relative contraindications to organ donation include age over 90 years, melanoma (except local melanoma treated more than 5 years before donation), disseminated cancer (above or below the diaphragm), and treated cancer within 3 years of donation (except nonmelanoma skin cancer and *in situ* cervical cancer).[222] Patients who die of disseminated chronic illness or multiorgan failure may potentially still donate their cornea or skin. Healthcare professionals are required by federal legislation to notify organ procurement organizations (OPOs) of all impending deaths.[226,227]

The timing of the discussion regarding organ donation is controversial, but in general, the issue should not be discussed until the family has come to the realization that the loved one is not going to survive. Best practice consists of the OPO and the healthcare team approaching the family together to discuss organ donation.[227] Palliative care can help with communication in several ways, including preparing the family for withdrawal of life support, aligning the different teams involved prior to organ harvesting, and educating and supporting families if involuntary movements are observed during withdrawal of life support.[222]

Organ donor cards (often found on the back of a driver's license) are legally binding. If a patient filled out an organ donor card, the family should not be asked about donation but told that their loved one wanted to donate.[227] Early contact with the OPO staff gives the patient and family time to discuss their concerns about organ donation such as logistics, cost, and time. The OPO staff is trained at effectively discussing these issues with families and providing appropriate psychosocial support.[227-230]

Ethics of Palliative and Hospice Care for Vulnerable Patients in Other Settings

According to the Institute of Medicine, "One of the greatest remaining challenges is the need for better understanding of the role of palliative care among both the public and professionals across the continuum of care so that hospice and palliative care can achieve their full potential for patients and their families."[231] Palliative care most often is provided in hospital-based palliative care consultation and outpatient hospice settings, but palliative care outpatient clinics are also becoming increasingly prevalent.[231] Nursing homes are a common site of death in the United States, yet much end-of-life care in nursing homes has been suboptimal, with inadequate pain control and transfers to acute care settings at the end of life.[232] Several barriers to quality end-of-life care in nursing homes have been identified, including communication between nursing home staff and family, pain management difficulties due to changing staff in the nursing home, and resident care issues.[233]

Hospice enrollment in nursing homes is associated with a higher quality of care than usual nursing home care.[234] Nursing home patients receiving hospice care are more likely to have pain assessed and treated, less likely to be hospitalized and die in a hospital, and less likely to have invasive treatment.[234] In addition to improvements in symptom relief, residents receiving hospice care have less fragmented care and are more likely to avoid hospitalization.[234] Quality of life of family members of hospice patients cared for in nursing homes was higher than quality of life of family members of hospice patients cared for in the community.[233] Nursing homes with more hospice use had lower risk of hospitalization for both hospice and nonhospice patients, suggesting that increased hospice presence may enhance quality of end-of-life care for all nursing home residents.[235]

In the past, financial disincentives existed that created barriers to hospice referral in nursing homes. Hospice is significantly more available in US nursing homes than palliative or comfort care programs,[236] and an increasing number of nursing home patients are using hospice, from 27.6% in 2004 to 39.8% in 2009, with increase in mean length of stay from 72.1 days to 92.6 days. Although there was less aggressive care at the end of life for nursing home residents from 2004 to 2009, there was an overall increase in Medicare expenditures during this period, likely due to the per diem reimbursement for hospice in patients with longer hospice stays.[237] For-profit hospices, which have grown from only 5% of hospices in 1990 to 51% of hospices in 2011, had longer mean length of stays, were more likely to exceed Medicare reimbursement limits, and had a higher patient disenrollment rate than nonprofit hospices in 2009.[238] Ongoing study will be needed to understand and optimize hospice and palliative care service delivery in the nursing home setting, as changes to the hospice benefit could decrease access to quality end-of-life care for nursing home residents.[239]

Providing Palliative Care in Challenging Situations

Care of the dying is challenging in the best of circumstances. When the patient is a child in an institutional setting or in foster care, an adult inmate in a prison, or a homeless person, it can be much more difficult. One example, the concept of prison hospice, demonstrates that the basic tenets of hospice care can be adapted to other settings. The large majority of dying prisoners do not have access to palliative care, but many facilities in the United States and United Kingdom have started hospice programs.[293] The five essential elements of prison hospice include: patient-centered care, inmate volunteer model, safety and security, shared values, and teamwork.[240] These programs often allow increased visitation, movement of prisoners within the prison, occasional amenities, and procedures for dispensing adequate amounts of pain medication.[294] Fellow prisoners are sometimes trained to function as a surrogate family for dying patients.[295] The National Prison Hospice Association[241] provides a collection of articles, videos and resources, and guidelines.[296]

According to the US Department of Housing and Urban Development, there has been an overall 11% decrease in the unsheltered homeless population since 2010, when President Barack Obama launched Opening Doors, the nation's first-ever comprehensive strategy to prevent and end homelessness.[297] Between 2010 and 2015, veteran homelessness declined 36%, family homelessness declined 19%, and chronic homelessness declined 22%.[297] Five factors are associated with increased risk of death for older homeless veterans: presence of a serious health issue, hospitalization for alcohol abuse, alcohol dependency, unemployment for 3 years, and age of 60 years and older.[242] Multiple programs have developed in response to the need to care for terminally ill homeless people, including Veteran Homestead; the Abbie Hunt Bryce Home in Indianapolis, IN; Mercy Hospice for the Homeless in Philadelphia, PA, and shelter-based palliative care programs.[243] However, the literature is currently limited on best practices and innovative models to care for these vulnerable patients. Many homeless individuals are estranged from family and friends, and thus are considered "unbefriended" (see Surrogate Decision Making on page 13).

Moral Distress

Clinical Situation

Mr. Garcia

Dr. Tucker, one of the hospital's palliative care attendings, receives a call from Nurse Ada on the medical floor. She asks if Dr. Tucker can come talk to Mrs. Garcia about her husband, who is currently hospitalized. She reports that Mr. Garcia is an 84-year-old man with dementia who was admitted from home with altered mental status. He has been diagnosed with aspiration pneumonia and a new stroke. Nurse Ada states that Mr. Garcia has a living will indicating that he did not want life-sustaining treatment if he was terminally ill.

She comments that Mr. Garcia's doctors are not painting a realistic picture when talking to Mrs. Garcia. She expresses concern because Mr. Garcia currently has a nasogastric feeding tube and needs restraints to keep it from being pulled out because of a hyperactive delirium. She comments that Mr. Garcia is suffering, is only going to get worse, and the care she is providing to him is only worsening his suffering. Nurse Ada comments, "I didn't go into nursing to torture people!"

From this short vignette, Nurse Ada appears to be very distressed about the situation. Dr. Tucker may recognize that Nurse Ada is suffering from moral distress. Moral distress occurs when clinicians believe that they know the right thing to do in a situation but are forced to do something different, which they believe is morally wrong. In the case of Mr. Garcia, Nurse Ada believes that using a feeding tube and restraining him are wrong. She believes that Mrs. Garcia is not being given accurate information about her husband's condition from the physicians. She believes that he wouldn't want the feeding tube because of what he wrote in his living will. She is new to her position and is not comfortable speaking up. Because she believes that the care this older man is receiving is morally wrong and she feels forced to be complicit in his care, we can empathize with her distress.

Numerous factors may increase the risk for development of moral distress. These factors include internal constraints (individual-based factors), external constraints (organization-based factors), and clinical causes (see **Table 9**). In examining cases of moral distress, although multiple clinicians may be experiencing moral distress from a given case, each clinician may be experiencing that distress due to different factors. In the case of Mr. Garcia, Nurse Ada may be experiencing moral distress because of her own inability to question what is being done, continuing care she does not believe is in Mr. Garcia's best interests and going against his preferences from his living will, and her belief that the physicians are providing Mrs. Garcia with false hopes about Mr. Garcia's chances of recovery.

With each case of moral distress encountered, a clinician's moral distress crescendos. When cases resolve, the clinician continues to have "moral residue," which increases over time.[244] One hypothesis is that "untreated" moral distress can lead to poor outcomes for patients, clinicians, and organizations.[245] When clinicians have moral distress, they may have difficulty advocating for their patients and may even have difficulties going into the patient's room, which may impact patient care. If clinicians find it increasingly difficult to care for certain patients because of their own moral distress, these clinicians may leave positions, or even leave their profession. Finally, for organizations in which staff moral distress is prevalent, certain units may experience high turnover and difficulties with retention of staff.

Palliative care clinicians may experience moral distress due to the cases they experience. They also may be consulted when other clinicians are experiencing moral distress. Those

Table 9. Risks for Moral Distress[244]

Internal constraints
- lack of assertiveness
- self-doubt
- socialization to follow orders
- perceived powerlessness
- lack of understanding of the full situation.

External constraints
- inadequate staffing
- hierarchies within the healthcare system
- lack of collegial relationships
- lack of administrative support
- policies and priorities that conflict with care needs
- compromised care due to pressure to reduce costs
- fear of litigation.

Clinical causes
- continue life support even though it is not in the best interest of the patient
- initiate lifesaving actions that only prolong death
- inappropriate use of resources
- continue aggressive care when no one will make the decision to discontinue life support
- work with physicians/nurses who are not as competent as care requires
- follow the family's wishes for the patient's care due to a fear of a lawsuit
- provide inadequate pain relief due to fear the increasing doses of pain medication will cause death
- provide false hope to patients and families.

From Moral distress, moral residue, and the crescendo effect, by EG Epstein and AB Hamric. J Clin Ethics. *2009;20(4):330-342. © 2009. All rights reserved. Reproduced with permission.*

suffering from moral distress may not recognize it as such. Palliative care clinicians can help their colleagues recognize and better understand moral distress.

Different interventions have been proposed to manage moral distress.[244,246-249] When intervening in situations of moral distress, it is important for all involved to understand the entire situation. For example, a team discussion about Mr. Garcia might ensure that all team members understand his medical condition. There may be a misunderstanding about his degree of dementia prior to his stroke. Other information about his condition that might be helpful for team members to know include 1) he had mild dementia and was independent with his ADLs prior to his stroke, 2) he has the potential for recovery of his swallowing function, and 3) he has a hyperactive delirium that is slowly resolving and contributing to his swallowing difficulties. Those caring for him also might learn that he was starved as a prisoner of war, and that his wife promised him that she would never allow this to happen to him again. With this additional information, clinicians might feel more hopeful about his situation and less concerned that they are providing him with inappropriate care.

Professional Boundaries[250]

Clinical Situation

Dr. Jennings

Dr. Jennings is conducting a palliative care consultation at the home of Mr. White, a 76-year-old man with end-stage COPD. Dr. Jennings has spent the last 1.5 hours hearing stories about Mr. White's nonconformist life. Mr. White reminds Dr. Jennings of her own grandfather. As she is finishing the visit, Mr. White asks if she would like to stay for dinner. She has enjoyed hearing his stories but is unsure if joining him for dinner is an appropriate thing to do.

When providing palliative care, clinicians often find themselves hearing intimate details of their patients' lives, and may even hear these details while in their patients' homes. For some clinicians, this situation can blur the boundaries between being a healthcare professional and being the patient's friend. When patients are considered and treated as friends, the clinician's objectivity and ability to provide quality care can be affected.

Professional boundaries are "mutually understood, unspoken physical and emotional limits" to the clinician-patient relationship.[251] Patients, especially those who have serious illness and are approaching the end of life, are potentially vulnerable. Clinicians have the knowledge and power to help their patients. In maintaining appropriate professional boundaries, clinicians remain aware of this power imbalance and do not act in ways that could potentially take advantage of patients. This improves patient care and also helps prevent clinician burnout.

During their careers, most clinicians cross one or more boundaries, either by mistake or in the spirit of patient care. Different types of boundary crossings exist (see **Table 10**). Boundary crossings are less serious and damaging to patients than boundary violations. For example, returning a hug from a patient is a boundary crossing, while engaging in a sexual relationship with a patient is a boundary violation. Clinicians should be mindful of boundary crossings because these may lead to boundary violations. Clinicians can ask themselves the questions in **Table 11** when questionable situations arise. Clinicians also may want to discuss questionable situations with trusted supervisors and/or colleagues. One way to decide about whether one is acting appropriately is to question whether the action is being taken for the good of the patient, or to meet the clinician's own needs.

Table 10. Boundaries in Patient-Physician Relationships

- Socialization with patients in person or via social media
- Dual relationships; employing patients you are also caring for
- Giving or receiving gifts
- Physical contact
- Self-disclosure
- Confidentiality and privacy of patient information

Table 11. Thinking About Whether My Action Crosses Professional Boundaries[250,252]

1. What are my institution's policies about this action (eg, receiving gifts or socializing with patients under my direct care)?
2. Does my profession address this action in its code of ethics?
3. What are the unique contextual features of this case?
4. Does the action respect my patient's autonomy and unique personhood?
5. Is the action for the benefit of my patient or to meet my own needs?
6. Could the action potentially harm my patient?
7. Am I treating this patient differently than my other patients? Why?
8. Am I being transparent about the action with others?
9. What would experienced colleagues or my clinical team say about the action?
10. What decisions or actions would my institution's ethics personnel consider ethically permissible or ethically forbidden?
11. How would I respond if it was written up in the local newspaper or posted on social media?

From The steak dinner—a professional boundary crossing, by EK Vig and MB Foglia. J Pain Symptom Manage. 2014;48(3):483-487. © 2014. All rights reserved. Reproduced with permission.

Informed Consent for Palliative Care Research

Increasing interest in outcome-based care is likely to generate much-needed research to help determine the efficacy of palliative interventions.[146,253] There are six ethical aspects of end-of-life care that should be considered when planning a research project or seeking approval from an institutional review board:

- whether the project is research or quality improvement
- potential benefit to future patients
- potential benefit to study subjects
- risks to study subjects
- subjects' decision-making capacity
- whether the subjects are freely volunteering to participate without significant controlling influences.[254]

Researchers should consider at least the basic issues of informed consent described in **Table 12**.[255,256] Informed consent issues should also be addressed when conducting research and reporting results.

Honest communication and adequate information are crucial to obtaining meaningful informed consent. The Nuremberg Code (1947) requires voluntary, competent, and informed consent to any medical procedure. The Declaration of Helsinki requires that adequate information be presented to potential research subjects and their family members about the aims of any research and its anticipated benefits and potential hazards.

Table 12. Basic Issues Related to Informed Consent in Research Settings[255,256]

Ongoing informed consent. Informed consent should be an ongoing process involving reevaluation as a patient's condition changes.

Cognitive ability. Determining a patient's cognitive ability to give informed consent is vital. When uncertain, researchers should use independent evaluators or instruments that measure cognitive ability. (See *UNIPAC 4* and *UNIPAC 9*.)

Surrogate permission. If a patient's mental incapacity precludes informed consent, surrogate consent is possible.

Risks and burdens. Full disclosure should be made to patients or their surrogates regarding the risks and burdens of participation, including the frequency and discomfort of invasive procedures, loss of privacy, and potentially burdensome expectations, such as completing daily logs and multiple questionnaires.

Patient's goals. Participating in research can provide dying patients with a renewed sense of purpose and a last opportunity to help others, but careful inquiry is needed to determine if this is truly the patient's goal or just the researcher's projected goal.

Recruitment. Recruiting an adequate number of participants is difficult because of the frequency of impaired mentation and emotional distress experienced by dying patients. Multisite projects often are necessary.

Roles of the clinician and the researcher. Patients are less likely to feel pressured to participate or to confuse the interests and goals of the researcher (completing the research project) with those of the clinician (caring for the patient) when the roles are separated.

Personal qualities of research personnel. When interacting with patients, data collectors and other research personnel should be particularly sensitive to the needs and vulnerabilities of seriously ill or dying patients and should discontinue research procedures when patients become fatigued or confused.

Reporting. Statements about consent are meaningless unless researchers include full descriptions of the methods used to obtain informed consent and the results are properly interpreted.

Final responsibility. No safeguards are more dependable than the presence of a responsible investigator who will ensure ethical conduct and protection of the rights of particularly vulnerable populations.

Obtaining informed consent in the research context is more problematic than in the clinical context. In the treatment context an intervention is intended to benefit the patient; in the research context the primary purpose of a study is to advance scientific knowledge and the intervention may not provide any patient benefit.[257] A patient may mistakenly believe that a proposed intervention will be beneficial and may be operating under a therapeutic misconception.[258] Such misconceptions are common in palliative care and elsewhere in medicine. This is particularly likely when a patient's treating physician is involved in the research study. Patients with terminal illnesses may feel compelled to participate under the mistaken notion that cure or life prolongation is possible or that the research is their only hope. In addition, these patients may feel obligated to participate in research to show their gratitude for care they are receiving, or they may be reluctant to withdraw from research that has become burdensome for fear they will be abandoned. Some patients under hospice and palliative care may be unable to withdraw from research because of rapid changes in cognitive capacity that limit their ability to reconsider participation.[129]

Most human subject research in the United States is governed by federal regulations—the common rules promulgated by the Department of Health and Human Services that are followed by several federal agencies and US Food and Drug Administration regulations.[259] Under these regulations the research protocol and consent document must be approved by an institutional review board.[260] Informed consent must be obtained from a research subject if he or she has decision-making capacity or, if the subject is incapacitated, from his or her legally authorized representative.[261] A surrogate who is authorized to make treatment decisions under state law also should be able to consent to participation in a research study.[146,258]

Despite the inherent difficulties of obtaining meaningful informed consent from terminally ill patients, research projects can be designed that heed the ethical considerations of nonmaleficence and patient autonomy and still provide much-needed information about the efficacy of palliative medicine interventions.[256,262] Proxy consent often is required, but, because a patient's ability to understand and express him- or herself can be volatile, a simple explanation of the procedures involved should be attempted in most situations. Facilitated consent, in which a close relative asks questions on behalf of the patient, but the actual consent is still provided by the patient, can enhance understanding and autonomy and is less burdensome.[263] It often is possible (and always desirable) to obtain assent for the protocol from compromised or underage patients (see AAHPM's position statement on Palliative Care Research on page 72 and *UNIPAC 7*).[264] Expressions of assent or dissent from participation must be respected even when proxy consent is obtained.[263]

AAHPM Statement on Palliative Care Research[265]

Approved by the AAHPM Board of Directors on November 4, 2014
(Replaces 2007 Palliative Care Research Ethics Joint Position Statement)

Background

Many palliative care decisions and interventions lack sufficient evidence to either recommend or not recommend. Much remains to be learned that could improve care of these patients, and further research in this field is needed. Debate exists about whether patients with serious illness should be asked to participate in research. Some clinicians, Institutional Review Boards (IRBs), ethics committees, and investigators remain uncertain about the ethical limits of research involving such patients and their families. IRBs have had limited guidance in reviewing palliative care protocols, and often their decisions vary widely. The principles of research ethics apply to all research, including palliative care research. The purpose of this document is to offer additional considerations to research on this potentially vulnerable patient population.

Statement

- Patients who receive palliative care should be considered for participation in clinical studies. Patients, regardless of where they are in their disease trajectory (impending death, difficult treatment regimens, complex diagnosis, etc.), should not be excluded from participation in clinical research.

- Research should be conducted with the informed consent of the patient, if possible, or surrogate decision maker. The choice to participate should always be voluntary.

- Uncertainty often exists around a serious or life-threatening illness. Researchers need to be sensitive to the patient situation, and should confer with the clinicians involved in the patient's care. Informed consent in this patient population may be a process rather than a one-time discussion as patient or study circumstances may change during the conduct of the research.

- Care should be taken to protect all patients and family, and especially the emotionally vulnerable, from therapeutic misconception (denial of the possibility of disadvantages of participation in clinical research related to the nature of the research process). Honesty about the benefits and burdens of participation in the study should be conveyed and understood by the patient.

- Mechanisms should be in place to refer research participants as needed (social services, clergy, bereavement specialists).

- Ideally, a palliative component should be included in clinical trials with patients whose diseases meet criteria for palliative medicine (eg, stage 4 cancer trials, COPD, end-stage liver disease, etc.) with a focus of the research on patient-centered outcome measures.

- If the researcher is the clinician for the patient, non-abandonment should be attached to the protocol. Continuity of care should be provided to these patients should they decide to withdraw from the research investigation.

Landmark Court Cases Relevant to Palliative Care

Palliative care is a fundamental part of end-of-life care, and although it focuses on the provision of care for pain and other symptoms, that provision also involves avoidance—of unwanted treatment. (How often have we heard someone say, "I don't want to be kept alive on machines"?)

Whereas treatment of severe symptoms and "existential suffering" often are challenging for the clinician to treat and hard for the patient to endure, by comparison it should be relatively simple for clinicians to prevent, and for patients to avoid, iatrogenic suffering. Iatrogenic suffering may fall on the most vulnerable patients, namely those who lack the capacity to make their own decisions and to "fight back." Those who have concerned relatives or others to advocate on their behalf have an advantage, but often the potential decision maker has insurmountable obstacles to act on the loved one's behalf.

It should not come as a surprise that only one of the termination-of-treatment cases discussed here involves a patient with a malignant disease.[266] Rather, the cases that have established legal precedent on refusal of treatment—the landmark cases—have almost always involved those with chronic diseases. Moreover, many are young; their age and condition permit long survival, long enough to attract attention, disagreement, frustration, and prolonged court proceedings, including those at the appellate level. One 1989 appellate case, not discussed here,[267] involved Larry McAfee, a 33-year-old competent patient with quadriplegia who wanted to receive sedation for terminal ventilator withdrawal. While enduring agonies over several years, his physicians refused to adequately sedate him for a terminal wean, perhaps for the reason that many physicians during that time refused to do this: on the basis that the medications would "kill" their patient and the physician would be held responsible. The court declared he had a right to be sedated during ventilator withdrawal, and the patient might have been so relieved by this that he decided to live.

The most tenacious arguments have focused on artificial nutrition and hydration (ANH), and decisions to discontinue ANH are fraught with emotion. Most landmark decisions on refusal of treatment have involved disagreements over tube feeding; in fact, five of the eight cases discussed here involved ANH. Although most appellate cases on which legal precedent is based have concerned young people with persistent vegetative state, most patients who actually receive long-term tube feeding have been elderly patients with advanced dementia.[268] Thus, the advocates, case history, and outcomes, may differ from what goes on in the "real world." Still, the lives of young people involved in the court cases have left behind victories for others.

Only one of the landmark cases discussed here involves a demand for treatment, the controversial case of Baby K, an anencephalic infant. The legal theory in this case was based on the Emergency Medical Treatment and Labor Act (EMTALA), the federal statute focusing on equal access to emergency medical treatment, and failed to advance the debate over medical "futility." One court case, not addressed here, was also not able to resolve the issue, at least not in the minds of clinicians and hospitals. This case involved Helga Wanglie,[269] an 87-year-old woman whose elderly spouse demanded treatment for her, but whose physicians unanimously considered her recovery hopeless and the situation frustrating. The court found, among other things, that the husband was the rightful decision maker. Despite the irony that this outcome may present for some, the case reiterated the right of family to make decisions, and the futility debate marches on.

Finally, as refusal-of-treatment cases have slowly faded into the background, the right to receive aid in dying came to the foreground. In both *Washington v Glucksberg* and *Vacco v Quill*, two cases heard by the US Supreme Court, terminally ill patients (all of whom had died by the time their cases reached the Court) wished to receive assistance in dying from their physicians, which was prohibited by law in their states. The Court did not find the laws to be unconstitutional, but left further decisions to the states to solve. As of this writing, the aid-in-dying movement continues to expand and evolve.

Quinlan (New Jersey Supreme Court, 1976)[270]

The Quinlan decision was the first to hold that the constitutional right of privacy, emanating from the concept of personal liberty, can be the basis for withholding or withdrawing mechanical life support in a person with no reasonable hope of recovery.

In 1975, when she was 21 years old, Karen Ann Quinlan suffered severe brain damage as the result of anoxia following accidental ingestion of a mixture of alcohol and prescription drugs. She was hospitalized and placed on mechanical ventilation and given ANH through a nasogastric tube. She remained unconscious, and her condition was eventually diagnosed as persistent vegetative state. Subsequently, her father sought court appointment as her guardian for the purpose of discontinuing "extraordinary medical treatment," namely, the respirator that was assisting her breathing, and which, when discontinued, would allow her to die. The treating physicians refused to discontinue the respirator, because this would not be in accord with medical standards. Mr. Quinlan's request to be appointed guardian was opposed by the treating physicians, the hospital, the local prosecutor, the State of New Jersey, and Karen's guardian ad litem. The trial court refused to appoint Mr. Quinlan as guardian of his daughter's person or authorize removal of the respirator. The Supreme Court of New Jersey reversed the trial court decision, thereby authorizing the withdrawal of life support and the appointment of Mr. Quinlan as guardian for that purpose if it was concluded, after appropriate consultation with a hospital ethics committee, that there was no reasonable possibility of Karen ever emerging from a persistent vegetative state.

The Supreme Court of New Jersey found that the right of Karen Ann Quinlan to refuse medical treatment, in this case to be exercised by her father as a surrogate, was protected by a right of privacy found in the federal and state constitutions, emanating from the constitutional concept of personal liberty. The court noted that the claimed interests of the state to preserve life and protect the right of physicians to administer treatment was in accordance with their best judgment, but that personal liberty overcomes that interest "when the degree of bodily invasion increases and the prognosis dims."[270]

The court endorsed the use of a substituted judgment standard—namely, allowing her guardian and family "to render their best judgment" regarding whether Karen would refuse the continuation of treatment if she were able. The court also endorsed the use of hospital ethics committees in reviewing decisions to withdraw life-sustaining treatment as preferable to court proceedings. It further concluded that the discontinuation of the respirator in this case would not result in criminal or civil liability.

The Quinlans were practicing Catholics and had been advised by their clergy that it would be permissible under Catholic teaching to discontinue the respirator, and their position had also been supported by a local Catholic bishop, who characterized the ventilator as "extraordinary treatment." The Supreme Court of New Jersey found that Catholic teaching was relevant insofar as it bore on the conscience of the proposed guardian.

Although she had spontaneous respiration shortly after hospital admission, she developed aspiration pneumonia the next day and she continued to require mechanical ventilation. During the first 6 months after her coma began, attempts to wean her from the ventilator failed, but over time she increasingly triggered the ventilator, and by the time of the high court's decision and subsequent ventilator withdrawal, she breathed on her own. Subsequently, the family did not seek to discontinue tube feeding or any other medical treatment, and Karen lived another 9 years. She died in 1985 from overwhelming systemic infection. Despite the expanded role for ethics committees envisioned in the *Quinlan* decision, the concept of hospital ethics committees did not immediately take hold, but are now widely endorsed and mandated for hospital accreditation.

Neuropathology of her autopsied brain revealed anoxic damage but unexpectedly revealed the greatest damage in the thalamus bilaterally, with only scattered areas of cerebrocortical damage.[271] This evaluation helped to pave the way for further analysis of the mechanisms behind cognition and arousal, and in the contemporary age of functional neuroimaging, the diagnosis of persistent vegetative state has been complicated by the identification of patients with "minimal states of consciousness."

Saikewicz (Supreme Judicial Court of Massachusetts, 1977)[266]

An early case that extended the right of a surrogate, in this case a court-appointed guardian, to make medical decisions for an adult with life-threatening illness who never had capacity. This case paved the way for additional attention to the needs of people with life-long intellectual disability (mental retardation) and related disorders of cognition.

On April 26, 1976, the superintendent of the Belchertown State School in Massachusetts requested a court to appoint a guardian to make medical decisions for Joseph Saikewicz, a 67-year-old resident of the school with an IQ of 10 and a mental age of 2 years and 8 months who had been institutionalized for 53 years. Saikewicz had been recently diagnosed with leukemia. The court appointed a guardian ad litem to make a recommendation on whether Saikewicz should receive treatment, and he recommended against it, saying it was not in the best interests of his ward. Saikewicz's treating physicians also recommended against treatment. Testimony at trial indicated there was a 30%–50% chance of remission, but typically remission only lasted 2 to 13 months. There also was testimony that chemotherapy was less likely to be successful in patients older than 60 years. The probate judge, agreeing with the guardian ad litem, ordered that no chemotherapy be administered, citing the incurable nature of the disease, the side effects connected with the treatments, and Saikewicz's inability to comprehend or cooperate with treatment.

The Supreme Judicial Court of Massachusetts affirmed holding that an incurably ill, incompetent patient acting through his or her guardian has the right to refuse life-prolonging treatment based on the common law doctrine of informed consent and the constitutional right of privacy. The court held that the substituted judgment standard applied in this case, noting:

> We believe that both the guardian ad litem in his recommendation and the judge in his decision should have attempted (as they did) to ascertain the incompetent person's actual interests and preferences. In short, the decision in cases such as this should be that which would be made by the incompetent person, if that person were competent, but taking into account the present and future incompetency of the individual as one of the factors which would necessarily enter into the decision-making process of the competent person. Having recognized the right of a competent person to make for himself the same decision as the court made in this case, the question is, do the facts on the record support the proposition that Saikewicz himself would have made the decision under the standard set forth. We believe they do.[266]

The Supreme Judicial Court further held that court involvement is necessary in nonemergent cases involving the withholding of life-sustaining treatment from incompetent patients. It stated that in such cases application should be made to a court for appointment of a guardian. In addition, the appellate court expressly rejected the suggestion made by the *Quinlan* court, discussed earlier, that review by an ethics committee in such cases is preferable to court proceedings. In yet another case (*Spring*), the Supreme Judicial Court of Massachusetts indicated that routine application to the courts in such cases may not be required to avoid civil liability.[272]

Although substituted judgment and certain other standards of decision making apply for persons who have lost capacity, such standards are controversial, or are seen as illogical, for someone who has never had capacity.[273] In the years since these decisions, legal procedures tailored to never-capacitated persons have evolved and are reviewed in the references.[274]

Barber (California Court of Appeal, 2nd District, 1983)[275]

In the first criminal prosecution for terminal withdrawal of life support with family consent, two physicians were charged with murder and conspiracy when their patient died. The Court determined "against a background of legal and moral considerations…of fairly recent vintage" that the death did not constitute murder and the family was permitted to decide for the patient. The court also considered ANH to be a treatment that could permissibly be withdrawn.

Two physicians, internist Neil Barber and surgeon Robert Nedjl, were charged with murder and conspiracy to commit murder when they withdrew life support at the request of the patient's family, after which the patient died. The patient, Clarence Herbert, had undergone a surgical ileostomy closure and suffered cardiac arrest while in the recovery room. He was resuscitated and placed on life support but remained comatose. After three days, physicians determined that he was unlikely to recover, and further evaluation by several consulting physicians determined that he had suffered severe brain damage and was in a vegetative state, which was not likely to resolve. The family was informed of the prognosis and repeatedly asserted their desire to have all life support discontinued. The patient breathed after ventilator withdrawal, and the family subsequently requested cessation of intravenous nutrition and hydration, after which the patient received nursing care until his death.

The charges initially were dismissed by a magistrate who held that the physicians' conduct was not the cause of the patient's death, and that the physicians had acted in good faith and in accordance with "ethical and sound medical judgment." The criminal complaint was reinstated by a California Superior Court judge who held that the physicians' intentional conduct shortened the patient's life and constituted murder under California law. The Superior Court judge also relied on the fact that the patient had not executed a living will under the California Natural Death Act. On appeal, a panel of the California Court of Appeal (the intermediate appellate court in California) held that the charges should be dismissed, finding that the execution of a living will under the California Death Act was not the exclusive method of making decisions to withdraw life-sustaining treatment. It also held that ANH should be viewed as medical treatment, that it was permissible to withdraw ANH without appointment of a legal guardian, and that the patient's wife and eight of their children, who had signed a written statement consenting to withdrawal, could act as surrogate decision makers. The panel noted that surrogate decision makers should apply a substituted judgment standard, but, even in the absence of evidence of the patient's wishes, ANH could be withdrawn under a best-interests approach when its burdens exceeded its benefits.

Conroy (Supreme Court of New Jersey, 1985)[276]

The case of Claire Conroy determined that patients who lack decisional capacity but are not in a vegetative state (such as those with severe dementia) may forgo life-sustaining treatments, including ANH. Although the court rejected the distinction between ANH and other life-sustaining treatments, it also complicated the traditional physician-family decision-making process with administrative procedures, sometimes requiring court intervention. Residents of nursing homes were deemed most vulnerable and additional procedures were required when refusal of life-sustaining treatment was sought in the nursing home setting.

The guardian and nephew of Claire Conroy, an 84-year-old nursing home resident, petitioned the court for approval to remove a nasogastric feeding tube that had been placed to provide her with long-term nutrition and hydration. Ms. Conroy suffered from advanced dementia and was not able to take sufficient nutrition or hydration by mouth, but she was not in a vegetative state. She was bedridden, with contractures, severe pressure sores, and a gangrenous leg. She was intermittently interactive and appeared able to experience discomfort, and sometimes smiled. Her nephew testified that she had never liked doctors and avoided them even if she was sick.

Because Conroy was Catholic, the trial court heard testimony from a Catholic professor of ethics at a seminary. He testified that, in light of Conroy's serious ailments and poor prognosis, the nasogastric tube could be considered extraordinary treatment. Accordingly, he opined that it would be ethical and moral to remove the tube. The trial court granted the nephew's request to withdraw the tube, finding that the burdens imposed by the treatment outweighed its benefits, but stayed its decision pending appeal by the guardian ad litem. During the appeal Conroy died, but the appellate division (the intermediate appellate court in New Jersey) decided the case because of the importance of the issues raised, and reversed the trial court, holding that removal of the nasogastric tube would be equivalent to active euthanasia.

The case then went to the Supreme Court of New Jersey, which reversed the appellate division, holding that even though Conroy was incapacitated, she had a right to refuse life-sustaining treatment (a right that could be exercised by her guardian under certain circumstances if proper precautions were followed), including ANH, which, it ruled, did not differ from other life-sustaining treatments. The court also outlined a series of procedures to be followed in patients who lack capacity.

The court first articulated a "subjective test," noting that evidence of what the patient would have wanted could be in a formal document such as a living will, in oral statements, or deduced from that person's religious or previous conduct with respect to medical treatment decisions. *Conroy* would not have satisfied the subjective test.

Even in the absence of such evidence, however, the court also recognized that the state could authorize guardians to terminate treatment under a best-interest approach, and further articulated two best-interest tests: "limited objective" and "pure objective." Satisfaction of either test could justify cessation of treatment. Under the limited objective test, treatment can be withheld "when there is some trustworthy evidence that the patient would have refused the treatment, and the decision maker is satisfied that it is clear that the burdens of the patient's continued life with the treatment outweigh the benefits of that life for him."[276] In the absence of "trustworthy evidence," treatment can be withdrawn under the pure objective test if "the net burdens of the patient's life with the treatment should clearly and markedly outweigh the benefits that the patient derives from life."[276]

The court further concluded, however, that incapacitated patients in nursing homes were entitled to additional procedural safeguards because of their special vulnerability. Thus, the court imposed three additional requirements applying to patients in nursing homes:

1. The patient must have been deemed incompetent to make the decision and must have a court-appointed guardian who is currently deemed to be the appropriate decision maker.
2. The State of New Jersey's Office of the Ombudsman for the Institutionalized Elderly must be notified of an intent to withdraw life-sustaining treatment and should process the matter as a possible case of "abuse," defined in the existing state statute as "a willful deprivation of services which are necessary to maintain a person's physical health."[277]
3. Two physicians not affiliated with the nursing home must be appointed and concur with the attending physician about the patient's condition and prognosis.

The court permitted withdrawal of treatment without court approval where the guardian, the two physicians, and the ombudsman concur that the subjective test, pure objective test, or limited objective test is satisfied. However, in *Conroy*, the court found that none of these tests were satisfied by the evidence adduced at trial.

Shortly after the *Conroy* decision, the state ombudsman issued a letter to all administrators of nursing homes and psychiatric hospitals in New Jersey, advising them that removal of ANH constituted abuse,[278] although the court in *Conroy* had explicitly noted that the definition of "abuse" pertaining to the ombudsman's oversight does not include withholding or withdrawing of ANH when the decision to do so has been appropriately addressed.[279] This letter created an outcry among physicians and others in New Jersey, leading to the resignation of the sitting ombudsman.

Bouvia (California Court of Appeal, 2nd District, 1986)[280]

This appellate case reaffirmed the right of a competent adult in California to refuse any medical treatment, including ANH and other life-sustaining treatments, even if the person is not "terminally ill" or "imminently dying."

Elizabeth Bouvia, at age 28, was a mentally competent woman who had been previously married and had obtained a college degree. She suffered from quadriplegia due to cerebral palsy at birth and was completely bedridden. She also had severe chronic pain due to arthritis, for which she received parenteral morphine. She was fed by spoon and ate as much as she could, stopping when she felt she could not eat more without nausea and vomiting. In the hospital, she was found to be very underweight, and a nasogastric feeding tube was inserted contrary to her instructions. She requested a court order to prohibit the continued use of tube feeding, but this was denied. The hospital maintained and the trial court concurred that such feeding was necessary to sustain life, that she intended to starve herself to death, and with adequate nutrition she could live another 15 to 20 years. The court refused to issue a preliminary injunction that would require removal of the feeding tube on the basis that the state's interest in the preservation of life outweighed her right to refuse treatment.

The case was appealed to the California Court of Appeal (the intermediate court level in the state), which reversed the lower court's decision. The court held that the "right to refuse medical treatment is basic and fundamental…recognized as a part of the right of privacy protected by both the state and federal constitutions…[and] its exercise requires no one's approval." The court furthermore clarified that a patient need not be "terminally ill" or "imminently dying" to exercise their right to refuse life-sustaining treatment, stating that the right exists "independent of the reason which may motivate the exercise of that right," and may do so even if those motives do not "meet with someone else's approval." Finally, it affirmed that a patient has the right to refuse any medical treatment or service, even when such treatment is labeled "furnishing nourishment and hydration," and even if exercising this right creates a "life threatening condition."[280]

Cruzan (United States Supreme Court, 1990)[37]

This was the first right-to-die case heard by the US Supreme Court. It established the right of competent persons to refuse life-sustaining treatment, including ANH, but permitted states to define standards of decision making for persons without capacity, including clear and convincing evidence, the highest evidentiary standards applied in civil cases.

In January 1983, Nancy Cruzan, a 25-year-old Missourian, was seriously injured in an automobile accident. When she was found lying face down, there was no detectable heartbeat or respiration. These functions were restored at the scene by paramedics, but at the hospital she remained unconscious. Physicians implanted a gastrostomy tube with permission of her then husband. Her condition subsequently was diagnosed as a persistent vegetative state.

Eventually, Cruzan's parents asked to have the tube feeding terminated, but hospital employees refused to accede to their request without a court order. The trial court recognized a constitutional right to refuse life-sustaining treatment and authorized withdrawal of ANH based upon its finding that before her injury, Cruzan had told a friend that if she were seriously injured she would not want to live unless she could live "halfway normally." The court found that these previous statements supported a desire to discontinue ANH, and not allowing her family to act on her behalf would deprive the patient of her rights under the law.

The hospital appealed, and the Supreme Court of Missouri reversed the decision of the trial court. Although the court recognized a right to refuse treatment under the common law doctrine of informed consent, it refused to recognize a constitutional right. It found a strong state interest in preservation of life as expressed in the Missouri Living Will Statute. On that basis, the court found that treatment could not be terminated in the absence of a valid living will unless it could be shown by "clear and convincing evidence" that the patient would have wanted it terminated. It found that the statements relied on by the trial court were unreliable and did not meet the clear and convincing evidence standard. The Cruzans then appealed to the US Supreme Court.

The US Supreme Court agreed to hear the case, and affirmed the decision of the Supreme Court of Missouri, holding that the state could require clear and convincing evidence of a person's expressed wishes made while competent. While the majority opinion upheld the constitutionality of the State of Missouri's requirement of clear and convincing evidence, it also acknowledged that "a constitutionally protected liberty interest in refusing unwanted medical treatment may be inferred from our prior decisions." The court stated, however, that because incompetent patients cannot exercise this right of refusal and need certain protections, it was appropriate for the State of Missouri to impose additional safeguards in the form of the clear and convincing evidence standard in light of its interest in preserving life (*Cruzan v Director*, 1990). The clear and convincing standard is the highest evidentiary standard that can be applied in a civil case.

After the Supreme Court decision, Nancy's family and friends found additional evidence of her previously expressed wishes, and the Cruzans petitioned the trial court in Missouri, again requesting discontinuation of tube feeding. Nancy's coworkers testified that she had stated she would not like to live "like a vegetable." Her treating physician and court-appointed guardian also supported discontinuation of ANH. This time, the trial court found there was clear and convincing evidence of Nancy's wishes. As a result of the new evidence, the Missouri court authorized the discontinuation of ANH and she died shortly thereafter, in December 1990.

The clear and convincing standard, permitted by the *Cruzan* decision, has been viewed by most clinicians as unrealistically stringent when applied in the clinical setting, when patients who lack capacity are dying and loved ones assert the person would not want to continue life support. Hence, the publicity surrounding this case fostered interest in advance directives, healthcare proxy appointments, and surrogate decision-making laws.

Baby K (US Court of Appeals, 4th Circuit, 1994)[281]

An infant born with anencephaly could be treated at the mother's insistence, despite the physician's judgment that treatment was medically inappropriate. Although sometimes viewed by clinicians as a "futility" case, the outcome hinged on the application of EMTALA, the federal statute requiring equitable treatment for all patients arriving at emergency rooms.

This case involved a Virginia infant who was born in 1992 with anencephaly, a condition in which parts of the brain, including the cerebral cortex, are missing. Babies with anencephaly lack higher-brain function, though autonomic functions are sustained by the brain stem. Medical standard of care at that time for such newborns consisted of the provision of supportive care (ie, nutrition, hydration, and warmth), and avoidance of aggressive measures, given the grave prognosis. Baby K's physicians recommended supportive care and discussed with the mother the possibility of entering a DNAR order. The mother rejected these recommendations and continued to insist that Baby K be provided with ventilator assistance when necessary.

The patient developed lung problems, and the mother insisted on treatment. The hospital was opposed to this and attempted to transfer the child but could not find another hospital to take the patient. The child was eventually transferred to a nursing home, where she developed repeated respiratory problems and apnea, leading to a number of transfers back to the hospital.

The hospital asked a US District Court to enter a judgment declaring that withholding ventilator treatment for Baby K, over the objection of her mother, would not violate the Emergency Medical Treatment and Active Labor Act (EMTALA). A federal statute, EMTALA requires hospitals that receive federal funds to screen any and all patients for an emergency medical condition and to provide stabilizing treatment to a patient such as this. EMTALA was crafted as an "antidumping" statute, seeking to prevent unequal treatment based on income or other patient factors that might be unappealing to providers, including a specific condition. The hospital argued that it was treating Baby K in the same way that it managed any other anencephalic infant, namely, by providing comfort care, and was therefore not violating EMTALA. The hospital also argued that EMTALA did not require them to provide ventilator treatment to Baby K because the treatment was futile and not in accordance with the prevailing medical standard of care. Furthermore, the hospital argued, under the Virginia Health Care Decisions Act (VHCDA), physicians can refuse to treat a patient whose surrogate insists on treatment that is "medically or ethically inappropriate."

The court rejected these arguments, stating, "EMTALA does not provide an exception for stabilizing treatment physicians may deem medically or ethically inappropriate." Furthermore, the VHCDA was designed to be applied in advance directive and surrogate decisions for adults, and not to decisions about infants.[281]

The District Court ruled against the hospital. On appeal, the US Court of Appeals affirmed, holding that under EMTALA the hospital had a duty to provide stabilizing treatment to Baby K when she arrived at the hospital in respiratory distress.

Baby K lived for 2.5 years, and her medical bills reportedly amounted to almost $1 million.[282] She eventually died at the hospital after being taken there for the sixth time by ambulance.

Washington v Glucksberg, Vacco v Quill (US Supreme Court, 1997)

In two cases appealed and heard together from 9th and 2nd federal circuit courts, the US Supreme Court unanimously ruled that the US Constitution does not guarantee the right to assisted suicide, and laws prohibiting assisted suicide may stand. Further debate on this issue was left to the states, leading to legalization of physician-assisted dying (PAD) in some states and stronger laws prohibiting PAD in certain others.

The US Supreme Court simultaneously heard cases that had been initiated in federal courts in New York and Washington state and appealed to the 2nd and 9th circuit courts, respectively. In these cases, patients who wished to obtain medication to end their lives, along with physicians and others, argued that laws in their respective states forbidding this practice violated their constitutional rights.

In New York state, three terminally ill patients and three physicians, including Dr. Timothy Quill, sued the State Attorneys General in the federal district court, arguing that New York's law banning assisted suicide violated the Equal Protection Clause of the 14th Amendment to the Constitution. In their argument, seriously ill, mentally competent patients who wish to have a physician's help to end their lives are no different from patients who require life support to stay alive; the latter have the right to end their lives by forgoing or discontinuing life support, but the former are not treated the same, even though their situation is arguably the same.

In Washington state, three terminally ill patients and four physicians, including Dr. Harold Glucksberg, along with a patient advocacy organization, sued in federal district court, asserting that the patients, who were competent and terminally ill, not only had a right under the Equal Protection clause, but also had a constitutionally protected liberty interest under the 14th Amendment Due Process clause, to obtain medication to end their lives.

The district court in New York disagreed with the equal protection argument, whereas the court in Washington agreed the patients had rights under both arguments. The cases were appealed to the 2nd and 9th circuits, respectively. Both circuit courts found that the state laws did violate the patients' rights and were unconstitutional, and the cases were appealed to the US Supreme Court. The Supreme Court disagreed with the circuit court holdings and reversed; thus, the states' bans on assisted suicide would stand.

With regard to the equal protection clause, the Court enumerated its previous recognition that "the distinction between letting a patient die and making that patient die…comports with fundamental legal principles of causation and intent…" that refusal of life-sustaining medical treatment results in death from the "underlying fatal condition…" whereas "if a patient ingests lethal medication prescribed by a physician he is killed by that medication."[108]

The Court also found that the due process clause was not violated; a liberty interest is protected if "deeply rooted in the nation's history," noting that in history and tradition, and contemporary law, assisted suicide has "never enjoyed legal protection similar to that protecting a person against unwanted touching."

In short, although guaranteeing the negative right to refuse unwanted treatment (see *Cruzan* case on page 80), the Constitution does not guarantee an affirmative right to obtain assistance in suicide, and existing laws in those states barring assisted suicide were not unconstitutional. Conversely, the Constitution does not explicitly forbid the practice. As the Court stated, "Americans are engaged in an earnest and profound debate about the morality, legality, and practicality of physician-assisted suicide. Our holding [reversing the decision of the Court of Appeals] permits this debate to continue, as it should in a democratic society."[187] To this end, as Supreme Court Justice O'Connor noted in her concurrence, the task is "entrusted to the 'laboratory' of the States…"

In addition to its holdings, the Court also distinguished assisted suicide from a hastened death resulting from "aggressive palliative care," such as administration of painkilling drugs for symptom control, which the state permits, and also seemed to specifically reject the claim that palliative sedation amounts to "covert physician-assisted suicide or euthanasia." Commentators have argued over whether these Supreme Court "dicta" indicate there is a constitutional right to palliative care,[195,283] but the practice of palliative sedation seems explicitly endorsed in both *Glucksberg*[187] and *Vacco*.[108]

In 1997, at the time of the Supreme Court's decision, all patients who had originally challenged their state laws had died. However, the holdings were followed by much legal activity in the states, including legalization of PAD in several states, on the one hand, as well as new or stronger state laws explicitly forbidding the practice on the other. As of this writing, PAD is prohibited by statute in a large majority of states. For further details, see Physician-Assisted Dying on page 53.

Schiavo (Florida, multiple courts)[284]

In the case of Terri Schiavo, a young woman in a persistent vegetative state, the patient's husband and her parents have a disagreement spanning over several years over the discontinuation of life-sustaining tube feeding. Court decisions repeatedly affirm the husband's decision to remove it. Called "perhaps the most thoroughly reviewed and litigated death in American history,"[285] this case involved not only multiple court hearings, but also intervention of the governor of Florida, US Congress, the president of the United States, and vocal input of "right-to-life" advocates, all in a background of papal statements on nutrition and hydration. The US Supreme Court refused to review the case. Fifteen years after the onset of her illness, the feeding tube was removed and Terri Schiavo died.

On February 25, 1990, at age 26, Theresa "Terri" Schiavo suffered cardiac arrest due to an extremely low potassium level linked to an eating disorder. She never regained consciousness, and eventually her condition was diagnosed as a persistent vegetative state. A feeding tube had been inserted to provide ANH.

Terri and her husband Michael had married in 1984. In 1990, he became Terri's court-appointed guardian, without the objection of Terri's parents, Robert and Mary Schindler. However, following malpractice settlement awards and disagreements about how the money was to be allocated, disagreements between Michael and the Schindlers ensued. Throughout Terri's illness, Michael's motivations and actions to pursue adequate medical care for Terri, including steps to find experimental therapy to try to reverse her condition, were undisputed, and his efforts continued despite other family disagreements. Finally, in 1998, he asked a Florida state trial court for permission to remove the feeding tube. At that time, it was clear that with ANH, Terri Schiavo could continue to live for many years. If it were withdrawn, she would die within a few days. The court granted permission after determining this was what Terri would have wanted, and authorized the withdrawal of ANH. The trial court's decision was affirmed by the Florida District Court of Appeals, which held that the trial judge had properly found under the clear and convincing evidence standard that Terri would have wanted the ANH discontinued.[284]

However, the Schindlers disagreed with the decision to remove the feeding tube and years of litigation followed.

The Florida courts had authorized the withdrawal of ANH after hearing much evidence about her previous statements as an adult. Schiavo and her family were Catholic, so Catholic teaching was an issue in the case, bearing on the question of what she would have wanted. In the original proceedings before the trial court, a Catholic priest from the Diocese of St. Petersburg, FL, testified regarding the Catholic Church's teaching on the withdrawal of ANH from patients in a persistent vegetative state. Schiavo's husband's attorney asked the priest whether removal of ANH would be consistent with the teaching of the Catholic Church. He further asked the priest to assume, for purposes of this question, that Terri Schiavo had told her husband she would not want to live "if she was dependent on the care of others" and moreover, that she "mentioned to her husband and to her brother and sister-in-law that she would not want to be kept alive artificially." The priest answered, "After all that has transpired, I believe, yes, it would be consistent with the teaching of the Catholic Church." On cross-examination, the priest was asked if he was familiar with Directive 58 in the 1994 Ethical and Religious Directives for Catholic Health Care Services, which states there should be a presumption in favor of providing ANH. He stated that he was familiar with Directive 58, but characterized it as providing an ideal standard, and further stated, "You have to go back and evaluate the proportion."[286] Schiavo's parents also attempted to convince the trial court that Terri was a practicing Catholic who was serious about her faith, but her husband testified that Terri was a lapsed Catholic. Ultimately, the courts looked to Terri's previous statements, finding clear and convincing evidence that Terri would have wanted the tube feeding removed. Ultimately the Florida appellate court sided with the husband, not only on the question of Theresa's religiosity but her other statements, and affirmed the trial court order permitting withdrawal of treatment.[284] The Schiavo case focused attention on Catholic teaching on withdrawal of ANH from patients in a persistent vegetative state and eventually resulted in a revision of Directive 58 (see the Catholic Healthcare Directives sidebar on page 44).

After the appellate court decision, additional legal wrangling continued for several years in both state and federal courts between her parents, who opposed removal of the feeding tube, and her husband, who sought its removal. The parents continued to contend that Terri was in a minimally conscious state rather than in a persistent vegetative state and that in light of her Catholic faith she would want the feeding continued. On October 15, 2003, Terri's feeding tube was removed.[284] Six days later, the Florida legislature passed a law allowing Governor Jeb Bush to order that the feeding be resumed. The feeding tube was reinserted, but this law subsequently was declared unconstitutional by the Florida Supreme Court.[287]

Terri Schiavo died on March 31, 2005, approximately 2 weeks after the removal of her feeding tube pursuant to a court order. After Terri's death, a neuropathological consultant's report accompanying the autopsy report confirmed the severity of the injuries to Terri's brain. Among other things, the report noted that the brain weight of 615 grams was only half of what was expected at her age, comparing this to the 835 gram brain at Karen Ann Quinlan's autopsy, whose clinical situation was comparable. However, the consultant's report noted that a neuropathological examination cannot determine whether the decedent had been in a persistent vegetative state before her death, as that is a "clinical examination arrived at through physical examination of living patients.[286] As in *Quinlan*, the *Schiavo* case focused additional attention on the evolving understanding of states of consciousness.[288,289] Furthermore, the unprecedented and unusual aspects of the *Schiavo* case raised a multitude of newer issues, including those of a cultural, religious, political, and ethical nature.[290,291]

References

1. Sugarman J, Sulmasy, DP (Eds.). *Methods in Medical Ethics (2nd ed.)*. Washington, DC: Georgetown University Press; 2010.

2. Jonsen AR, Siegler M, Winslade WJ. *Clinical Ethics: A Practical Approach to Ethical Decisions in Clinical Medicine*. 7th ed. New York, NY: McGraw-Hill; 2010.

3. Kaldjian LC, Weir RF, Duffy TP. A clinician's approach to clinical ethical reasoning. *J Gen Intern Med*. 2005;20(3):306-311.

4. Berkowitz KA, Chanko BL, Foglia MB, Fox E, Powell T. National Center for Ethics in Health Care, Ethics Consultation: Responding to Ethics Questions in Health Care. 2nd ed. Washington, DC: U.S. Department of Veterans Affairs; 2015.

5. Periyakoil VS, Neri E, Fong A, Kraemer H. Do unto others: doctors' personal end-of-life resuscitation preferences and their attitudes toward advance directives. *PloS One*. 2014;9(5):e98246.

6. Ubel PA, Angott AM, Zikmund-Fisher BJ. Physicians recommend different treatments for patients than they would choose for themselves. *Arch Intern Med*. 2011;171(7):630-634.

7. Pellegrino ED. Toward a virtue-based normative ethics for the health professions. *Kennedy Inst Ethics J*. 1995;5(3):253-277.

8. Jeffery P, Millard PH. An ethical framework for clinical decision-making at the end of life. *J R Soc Med*. 1997;90(9):504-506.

9. Silveira MJ, Kim SY, Langa KM. Advance directives and outcomes of surrogate decision making before death. *N Engl J Med*. 2010;362(13):1211-1218.

10. Bosslet GT, Pope TM, Rubenfeld GD, et al. An Official ATS/AACN/ACCP/ESICM/SCCM Policy Statement: Responding to Requests for Potentially Inappropriate Treatments in Intensive Care Units. *Am J Respir Crit Care Med*. 2015;191(11):1318-1330.

11. Legare F, Stacey D, Turcotte S, et al. Interventions for improving the adoption of shared decision making by healthcare professionals. *Cochrane Database Syst Rev*. 2014(9):Cd006732.

12. Stacey D, Bennett CL, Barry MJ, et al. Decision aids for people facing health treatment or screening decisions. *Cochrane Database Syst Rev*. 2011(10):CD001431.

13. Grady C. Enduring and emerging challenges of informed consent. *N Engl J Med*. 2015;372(9):855-862.

14. Kinnersley P, Phillips K, Savage K, et al. Interventions to promote informed consent for patients undergoing surgical and other invasive healthcare procedures. *Cochrane Database Syst Rev*. 2013(7):Cd009445.

15. Weissman DE, Derse A. Informed consent in palliative care: part I #164. *J Palliat Med*. 2011;14(9):1065-1066.

16. Nelson LJ. Consent to treatment. Vol in David W. Louisell and Harold Williams, Medical Malpractice § 22.05 2011.

17. American Medical Association. Informed consent. www.ama-assn.org/ama/pub/category/4608.html. Accessed August 3, 2007.

18. Ganzini L, Volicer L, Nelson WA, Fox E, Derse AR. Ten myths about decision-making capacity. *J Am Med Dir Assoc*. 2004;5(4):263-267.

19. Miller SS, Marin DB. Assessing capacity. *Emerg Med Clin North Am*. 2000;18(2):233-242.

20. Hastings Center. *Guidelines on the Termination of Life-Sustaining Treatment and the Care of the Dying: A Report*. Bloomington, IN: Indiana University Press; 1987.

21. Scott JF, Lynch J. Bedside assessment of competency in palliative care. *J Palliat Care*. 1994;10(3):101-105.

22. Duncan E, Best C, Hagen S. Shared decision making interventions for people with mental health conditions. *Cochrane Database Syst Rev*. 2010(1):CD007297.

23. Hamann J, Bronner K, Margull J, et al. Patient participation in medical and social decisions in Alzheimer's disease. *J Am Geriatr Soc.* 2011;59(11):2045-2052.

24. Chow GV, Czarny MJ, Hughes MT, Carrese JA. CURVES: a mnemonic for determining medical decision-making capacity and providing emergency treatment in the acute setting. *Chest.* 2010;137(2):421-427.

25. Etchells E, Darzins P, Silberfeld M, et al. Assessment of patient capacity to consent to treatment. *J Gen Intern Med.* 1999;14(1):27-34.

26. Sessums LL, Zembrzuska H, Jackson JL. Does this patient have medical decision-making capacity? *JAMA.* 2011;306(4):420-427.

27. Etchells E. Aid to capacity evaluation (ACE). http://www.jcb.utoronto.ca/tools/documents/ace.pdf. Accessed June 27, 2016.

28. Fazel S, Hope T, Jacoby R. Assessment of competence to complete advance directives: validation of a patient centred approach. *BMJ.* 1999;318(7182):493-497.

29. Luce JM. End-of-life decision making in the intensive care unit. *Am J Respir Crit Care Med.* 2010;182(1):6-11.

30. Pope TM. The best interest standard: both guide and limit to medical decision making on behalf of incapacitated patients. *J Clin Ethics.* 2011;22(2):134-138.

31. Default surrogate consent statutes. 2014; http://www.americanbar.org/content/dam/aba/administrative/law_aging/2014_default_surrogate_consent_statutes.authcheckdam.pdf Accessed June 30, 2016.

32. American Bar Association. Health Care Decision-Making. http://www.americanbar.org/groups/law_aging/resources/health_care_decision_making.html.

33. Beauchamp TL, Childress JF. *Principles of Biomedical Ethics.* 6th ed. New York: Oxford University Press; 2009.

34. Farrell TW, Widera E, Rosenberg L, et al. AGS position statement: making medical treatment decisions for unbefriended older adults. *J Am Geriatr Soc.* 2016.

35. Meisel A, Cerminara KL. *Right to Die: The Law of End-of-Life Decision Making.* 3rd ed. Riverwoods, IL: Aspen Publishers; 2011.

36. Edwards SJ, Brown P, Twyman MA, Christie D, Rakow T. A qualitative investigation of selecting surrogate decision-makers. *J Med Ethics.* 2011;37(10):601-605.

37. *Cruzan v Director, Missouri Department of Health,* 497 US 261 (1990).

38. Shalowitz DI, Garrett-Mayer E, Wendler D. The accuracy of surrogate decision makers: a systematic review. *Arch Intern Med.* 2006;166(5):493-497.

39. Gilmour J, Harrison C, Asadi L, Cohen MH, Aung S, Vohra S. Considering complementary and alternative medicine alternatives in cases of life-threatening illness: applying the best-interests test. *Pediatrics.* 2011;128 Suppl 4:S175-180.

40. McLennan S. CPR policies and the patient's best interests. *Resuscitation.* 2011.

41. Vig EK, Taylor JS, Starks H, Hopley EK, Fryer-Edwards K. Beyond substituted judgment: how surrogates navigate end-of-life decision-making. *J Am Geriatr Soc.* 2006;54(11):1688-1693.

42. Sulmasy DP, Snyder L. Substituted interests and best judgments: an integrated model of surrogate decision making. *JAMA.* 2010;304(17):1946-1947.

43. Bruce CR, Bibler T, Childress AM, Stephens AL, Pena AM, Allen NG. Navigating ethical conflicts between advance directives and surrogate decision-makers' interpretations of patient wishes. *Chest.* 2016;149(2):562-567.

44. Vig EK, Sudore RL, Berg KM, Fromme EK, Arnold RM. Responding to surrogate requests that seem inconsistent with a patient's living will. *J Pain Symptom Manage.* 2011;42(5):777-782.

45. Sudore RL. A piece of my mind. Can we agree to disagree? *JAMA.* 2009;302(15):1629-1630.

46. Brush DR, Brown CE, Alexander GC. Critical care physicians' approaches to negotiating with surrogate decisionmakers: a qualitative study. *Crit Care Med.* 2011.

47. Kinzbrunner BM. Jewish medical ethics and end-of-life care. *J Palliat Med.* 2004;7(4):558-573.

48. Baeke G, Wils JP, Broeckaert B. Orthodox Jewish perspectives on withholding and withdrawing life-sustaining treatment. *Nurs Ethics.* 2011;18(6):835-846.

49. Sterilization or Abortion Act, 42 USC, §300a-7 (1973).

50. Public Welfare: Definitions. To be codified at 45 CFR §88.2. *Fed Registr.* 2008;73:414-415.

51. State Plans for Medical Assistance Act, 42 USC, §1395-1396 (2011).

52. Mueller LA, Reid KI, Mueller PS. Readability of state-sponsored advance directive forms in the United States: a cross sectional study. *BMC Med Ethics.* 2010;11:6.

53. Mirarchi FL, Costello E, Puller J, Cooney T, Kottkamp N. TRIAD III: nationwide assessment of living wills and do not resuscitate orders. *J Emerg Med.* 2011.

54. Levi BH, Heverley SR, Green MJ. Accuracy of a decision aid for advance care planning: simulated end-of-life decision making. *J Clin Ethics.* 2011;22(3):223-238.

55. Tunzi M. Advance care directives: realities and challenges in central California. *J Clin Ethics.* 2011;22(3):239-248.

56. Garand L, Dew MA, Lingler JH, DeKosky ST. Incidence and predictors of advance care planning among persons with cognitive impairment. *Am J Geriatr Psychiatry.* 2011;19(8):712-720.

57. Sizoo EM, Pasman HR, Buttolo J, et al. Decision-making in the end-of-life phase of high-grade glioma patients. *Eur J Cancer.* 2012;48(2):226-232.

58. Tan TS, Jatoi A. End-of-life hospital costs in cancer patients: do advance directives or routes of hospital admission make a difference? *Oncology.* 2011;80(1-2):118-122.

59. Silveira MJ, DiPiero A, Gerrity MS, Feudtner C. Patients' knowledge of options at the end of life: ignorance in the face of death. *JAMA.* 2000;284(19):2483-2488.

60. Singer PA. Advance directives in palliative care. *J Palliat Care.* 1994;10(3):111-116.

61. Briggs L. Shifting the focus of advance care planning: using an in-depth interview to build and strengthen relationships. *Innovations in End-of-Life Care.* 2003;5(2). www.edc.org/lastacts. Accessed August 3, 2007.

62. Houben CH, Spruit MA, Groenen MT, Wouters EF, Janssen DJ. Efficacy of advance care planning: a systematic review and meta-analysis. *J Am Med Dir Assoc.* 2014;15(7):477-489.

63. Nicholas LH, Langa KM, Iwashyna TJ, Weir DR. Regional variation in the association between advance directives and end-of-life Medicare expenditures. *JAMA.* 2011;306(13):1447-1453.

64. Hackler JC, Hiller FC. Family consent to orders not resuscitate. Reconsidering hospital policy. *JAMA.* 1990;264(10):1281-1283.

65. Blackhall LJ. Must we always use CPR? *N Engl J Med.* 1987;317(20):1281-1285.

66. Yuen JK, Reid MC, Fetters MD. Hospital do-not-resuscitate orders: why they have failed and how to fix them. *J Gen Intern Med.* 2011;26(7):791-797.

67. Kaldjian LC, Erekson ZD, Haberle TH, et al. Code status discussions and goals of care among hospitalised adults. *J Med Ethics.* 2009;35(6):338-342.

68. Neagle JT, Wachsberg K. What are the chances a hospitalized patient will survive in-hospital arrest? *The Hospitalist.* 2010; http://www.the-hospitalist.org/hospitalist/article/124220/what-are-chances-hospitalized-patient-will-survive-hospital-arrest.

69. Tian J, Kaufman DA, Zarich S, et al. Outcomes of critically ill patients who received cardiopulmonary resuscitation. *Am J Respir Crit Care Med.* 2010;182(4):501-506.

70. Wong SP, Kreuter W, Curtis JR, Hall YN, O'Hare AM. Trends in in-hospital cardiopulmonary resuscitation and survival in adults receiving maintenance dialysis. *JAMA Intern Med.* 2015;175(6):1028-1035.

71. Reisfield GM, Wallace SK, Munsell MF, Webb FJ, Alvarez ER, Wilson GR. Survival in cancer patients undergoing in-hospital cardiopulmonary resuscitation: a meta-analysis. *Resuscitation.* 2006;71(2):152-160.

72. Finucane TE, Harper M. Ethical decision-making near the end of life. *Clin Geriatr Med.* 1996;12(2):369-377.

73. Bruera E, Neumann CM, Mazzocato C, Stiefel F, Sala R. Attitudes and beliefs of palliative care physicians regarding communication with terminally ill cancer patients. *Palliat Med.* 2000;14(4):287-298.

74. Dzeng E, Colaianni A, Roland M, et al. Influence of institutional culture and policies on do-not-resuscitate decision making at the end of life. *JAMA Intern Med.* 2015;175(5):812-819.

75. Cardenas-Turanzas M, Gaeta S, Ashoori A, Price KJ, Nates JL. Demographic and clinical determinants of having do not resuscitate orders in the intensive care unit of a comprehensive cancer center. *J Palliat Med.* 2011;14(1):45-50.

76. Parsons HA, de la Cruz MJ, Zhukovsky DS, et al. Characteristics of patients who refuse do-not-resuscitate orders upon admission to an acute palliative care unit in a comprehensive cancer center. *Cancer.* 2010;116(12):3061-3070.

77. National Hospice Organization. *Do Not Resuscitate (DNAR) Decisions in the Context of Hospice Care.* Arlington, VA: National Hospice Organization; 1992.

78. Alpers A, Lo B. When is CPR futile? *JAMA.* 1995;273(2):156-158.

79. von Gunten CF. Discussing do-not-resuscitate status. *J Clin Oncol.* 2001;19(5):1576-1581.

80. Delisser HM. A practical approach to the family that expects a miracle. *Chest.* 2009;135(6):1643-1647.

81. Widera EW, Rosenfeld KE, Fromme EK, Sulmasy DP, Arnold RM. Approaching patients and family members who hope for a miracle. *J Pain Symptom Manage.* 2011;42(1):119-125.

82. Saager L, Kurz A, Deogaonkar A, et al. Pre-existing do-not-resuscitate orders are not associated with increased postoperative morbidity at 30 days in surgical patients. *Crit Care Med.* 2011;39(5):1036-1041.

83. Quill TE, Arnold R, Back AL. Discussing treatment preferences with patients who want "everything." *Ann Intern Med.* 2009;151(5):345-349.

84. Truog RD. Is it always wrong to perform futile CPR? *N Engl J Med.* 2010;362(6):477-479.

85. Lee MD, Friedenberg AS, Mukpo DH, Conray K, Palmisciano A, Levy MM. Visiting hours policies in New England intensive care units: strategies for improvement. *Crit Care Med.* 2007;35(2):497-501.

86. Kosowan S, Jensen L. Family presence during cardiopulmonary resuscitation: cardiac health care professionals' perspectives. *Can J Cardiovasc Nurs.* 2011;21(3):23-29.

87. Jabre P, Belpomme V, Azoulay E, et al. Family presence during cardiopulmonary resuscitation. *N Engl J Med.* 2013;368(11):1008-1018.

88. Hickman SE, Keevern E, Hammes BJ. Use of the physician orders for life-sustaining treatment program in the clinical setting: a systematic review of the literature. *J Am Geriatr Soc.* 2015;63(2):341-350.

89. Breuer B, Fleishman SB, Cruciani RA, Portenoy RK. Medical oncologists' attitudes and practice in cancer pain management: a national survey. *J Clin Oncol.* 2011;29(36):4769-4775.

90. Jacox A, Carr DB, Payne R, et al. *Management of Cancer Pain. Clinical Practice Guideline No. 9.* Rockville, MD: Agency for Health Care Policy and Research, US Department of Health and Human Services; 1994.

91. Glajchen M. Chronic pain: treatment barriers and strategies for clinical practice. *J Am Board Fam Pract.* 2001;14(3):211-218.

92. Sullivan M. Ethical principles in pain management. *Pain medicine (Malden, Mass.).* 2001;2(2):106-111.

93. Billings JA. Double effect: a useful rule that alone cannot justify hastening death. *J Med Ethics.* 2011;37(7):437-440.

94. El-Jawahri A, Greer JA, Temel JS. Does palliative care improve outcomes for patients with incurable illness? A review of the evidence. *J Support Oncol.* 2011;9(3):87-94.

95. Temel JS, Greer JA, Muzikansky A, et al. Early palliative care for patients with metastatic non-small-cell lung cancer. *N Engl J Med.* 2010;363(8):733-742.

96. Quill TE, Dresser R, Brock DW. The rule of double effect—a critique of its role in end-of-life decision making. *N Engl J Med.* 1997;337(24):1768-1771.

97. Institute for Healthcare Improvement. The IHI Triple Arm. http://www.ihi.org/Engage/Initiatives/TripleAim/Pages/default.aspx. Accessed May 30, 2017.

98. Snyder L, American College of Physicians. *Ethics Manual.* 6th ed. Philadelphia, PA: American College of Physicians; 2012.

99. Truog RD, Brett AS, Frader J. The problem with futility. *N Engl J Med.* 1992;326(23):1560-1564.

100. Schneiderman LJ, Jecker NS, Jonsen AR. Medical futility: its meaning and ethical implications. *Ann Intern Med.* 1990;112(12):949-954.

101. Rebagliato M, Cuttini M, Broggin L, et al. Neonatal end-of-life decision making: physicians' attitudes and relationship with self-reported practices in 10 European countries. *JAMA.* 2000;284(19):2451-2459.

102. Bernat JL. Medical futility: definition, determination, and disputes in critical care. *Neurocrit Care.* 2005;2(2):198-205.

103. Procedure if Not Effectuating a Directive or Treatment Decision, Tex. Health & Safety Code, §166.046 (2003).

104. Burge CR. Texas Advance Directives Act versus "state-created danger" theory: a prima facie analysis. *Am J Trial Advoc.* 2009;32:552.

105. Fine RL. Point: the Texas advance directives act effectively and ethically resolves disputes about medical futility. *Chest.* 2009;136(4):963-967.

106. Truog RD. Counterpoint: the Texas advance directives act is ethically flawed: medical futility disputes must be resolved by a fair process. *Chest.* 2009;136(4):968-971.

107. Shannon S. Medical futility and professional integrity, religious tolerance, and social justice. *ASBH Exchange.* 2006(Spring):9-10.

108. *Vacco v Quill,* 521 US 793, 807 (1997).

109. Cohen AB, Wright MS, Cooney L Jr., Fried T. Guardianship and end-of-life decision making. *JAMA Intern Med.* 2015;175(10):1687-1691.

110. Sulmasy DP. Speaking of the value of life. *Kennedy Inst Ethics J.* 2011;21(2):181-199.

111. Christakis NA, Asch DA. Biases in how physicians choose to withdraw life support. *Lancet.* 1993;342(8872):642-646.

112. University of Washington School of Medicine. Termination of Life-Sustaining Treatment. http://depts.washington.edu/bioethx/topics/termlife.html. Accessed January 12, 2012.

113. Rydvall A, Lynoe N. Withholding and withdrawing life-sustaining treatment: a comparative study of the ethical reasoning of physicians and the general public. *Crit Care.* 2008;12(1):R13.

114. Quill TE, Holloway R. Time-limited trials near the end of life. *JAMA.* 2011;306(13):1483-1484.

115. National Council for Hospice and Specialist Palliative Care Services. *Key Ethical Issues in Palliative Care: Evidence to House of Lords Select Committee on Medical Ethics.* London, UK: National Council for Hospice and Specialist Palliative Care Services; 1993.

116. Curtis JR, Vincent JL. Ethics and end-of-life care for adults in the intensive care unit. *Lancet.* 2010;376(9749):1347-1353.

117. Karches KE, Sulmasy DP. Ethical considerations for turning off pacemakers and defibrillators. *Card Electrophysiol Clin.* 2015;7(3):547-555.

118. Schmidt TA, Hickman SE, Tolle SW, Brooks HS. The Physician Orders for Life-Sustaining Treatment program: Oregon emergency medical technicians' practical experiences and attitudes. *J Am Geriatr Soc.* 2004;52(9):1430-1434.

119. Johnson J, Hayden T, True J, et al. The impact of faith beliefs on perceptions of end-of-life care and decision making among African American church members. *J Palliat Med.* 2016;19(2):143-148.

120. Smith-Howell ER, Hickman SE, Meghani SH, Perkins SM, Rawl SM. End-of-life decision making and communication of bereaved family members of African Americans with serious illness. *J Palliat Med.* 2016;19(2):174-182.

121. Mitchell BL, Mitchell LC. Review of the literature on cultural competence and end-of-life treatment decisions: the role of the hospitalist. *J Natl Med Assoc.* 2009;101(9):920-926.

122. Hazin R, Giles CA. Is there a color line in death? An examination of end-of-life care in the African American community. *J Natl Med Assoc.* 2011;103(7):609-613.

123. Foronda C, Baptiste DL, Reinholdt MM, Ousman K. Cultural humility: a concept analysis. *J Transcult Nurs.* 2016;27(3):210-217.

124. American Academy of Hospice and Palliative Medicine. AAHPM Position Statement on Withholding and Withdrawing Non Beneficial Medical Interventions. http://aahpm.org/positions/withholding-nonbeneficial-interventions. Accessed January 11, 2012.

125. American Geriatrics Society feeding tubes in advanced dementia position statement. *J Am Geriatr Soc.* 2014;62(8):1590-1593.

126. Good P, Richard R, Syrmis W, Jenkins-Marsh S, Stephens J. Medically assisted hydration for adult palliative care patients. *Cochrane Database Syst Rev.* 2014(4):Cd006273.

127. Good P, Richard R, Syrmis W, Jenkins-Marsh S, Stephens J. Medically assisted nutrition for adult palliative care patients. *Cochrane Database Syst Rev.* 2014(4):Cd006274.

128. Teno JM, Gozalo PL, Mitchell SL, et al. Does feeding tube insertion and its timing improve survival? *J Am Geriatr Soc.* 2012;60(10):1918-1921.

129. Hall S, Longhurst S, Higginson IJ. Challenges to conducting research with older people living in nursing homes. *BMC Geriatr.* 2009;9:38.

130. Goold SD, Williams B, Arnold RM. Conflicts regarding decisions to limit treatment: a differential diagnosis. *JAMA.* 2000;283(7):909-914.

131. Meier DE, Ahronheim JC, Morris J, Baskin-Lyons S, Morrison RS. High short-term mortality in hospitalized patients with advanced dementia: lack of benefit of tube feeding. *Arch Intern Med.* 2001;161(4):594-599.

132. Teno JM, Gozalo P, Mitchell SL, Kuo S, Fulton AT, Mor V. Feeding tubes and the prevention or healing of pressure ulcers. *Arch Intern Med.* 2012;172(9):697-701.

133. Givens JL, Selby K, Goldfeld KS, Mitchell SL. Hospital transfers of nursing home residents with advanced dementia. *J Am Geriatr Soc.* 2012;60(5):905-909.

134. Mitchell SL, Teno JM, Kiely DK, et al. The clinical course of advanced dementia. *N Engl J Med.* 2009;361(16):1529-1538.

135. American Academy of Hospice and Palliative Medicine. Five Things Physicians and Patients Should Question. 2013; http://www.choosingwisely.org/societies/american-academy-of-hospice-and-palliative-medicine/. Accessed May 31, 2017.

136. Gillick MR. Rethinking the role of tube feeding in patients with advanced dementia. *N Engl J Med.* 2000;342(3):206-210.

137. Good P, Cavenagh J, Mather M, Ravenscroft P. Medically assisted hydration for palliative care patients. *Cochrane Database Syst Rev.* 2008(2):CD006273.

138. Ganzini L, Goy ER, Miller LL, Harvath TA, Jackson A, Delorit MA. Nurses' experiences with hospice patients who refuse food and fluids to hasten death. *N Engl J Med.* 2003;349(4):359-365.

139. Fuhrman MP, Herrmann VM. Bridging the continuum: nutrition support in palliative and hospice care. *Nutr Clin Pract.* 2006;21(2):134-141.

140. Hui D, Dev R, Bruera E. The last days of life: symptom burden and impact on nutrition and hydration in cancer patients. *Curr Opin Support Palliat Care.* 2015;9(4):346-354.

141. Chermesh I, Mashiach T, Amit A, et al. Home parenteral nutrition (HTPN) for incurable patients with cancer with gastrointestinal obstruction: do the benefits outweigh the risks? *Med Oncol.* 2011;28(1):83-88.

142. United States Conference of Catholic Bishops. Ethical and Religious Directives for Catholic Health Care Services. 5th ed. http://www.ncbcenter.org/document.doc?id=147. Accessed January 11, 2012.

143. Druml C, Ballmer PE, Druml W, et al. ESPEN guideline on ethical aspects of artificial nutrition and hydration. *Clin Nutr.* 2016;35(3):545-556.

144. Preston T, Kelly M. A medical ethics assessment of the case of Terri Schiavo. *Death Stud.* 2006;30(2):121-133.

145. Thomas DR, Cote TR, Lawhorne L, et al. Understanding clinical dehydration and its treatment. *J Am Med Dir Assoc.* 2008;9(5):292-301.

146. Csikai EL. Developing the science of end-of-life and palliative care research: National Institute of Nursing Research Summit. *J Soc Work End Life Palliat Care.* 2011;7(4):291-299.

147. McCann RM, Hall WJ, Groth-Juncker A. Comfort care for terminally ill patients. The appropriate use of nutrition and hydration. *JAMA.* 1994;272(16):1263-1266.

148. Bruera E, Hui D, Dalal S, et al. Parenteral hydration in patients with advanced cancer: a multicenter, double-blind, placebo-controlled randomized trial. *J Clin Oncol.* 2013;31(1):111-118.

149. Gillick MR. The use of advance care planning to guide decisions about artificial nutrition and hydration. *Nutr Clin Pract.* 2006;21(2):126-133.

150. Tresch DD, Sims FH, Duthie EH, Jr., Goldstein MD. Patients in a persistent vegetative state attitudes and reactions of family members. *J Am Geriatr Soc.* 1991;39(1):17-21.

151. Ciocon JO, Silverstone FA, Graver LM, Foley CJ. Tube feedings in elderly patients. Indications, benefits, and complications. *Arch Intern Med.* 1988;148(2):429-433.

152. Bozzetti F, Arends J, Lundholm K, Micklewright A, Zurcher G, Muscaritoli M. ESPEN guidelines on parenteral nutrition: nonsurgical oncology. *Clin Nutr.* 2009;28(4):445-454.

153. American Academy of Hospice and Palliative Medicine. AAHPM Statement on Artificial Nutrition and Hydration Near the End of Life. http://aahpm.org/positions/anh. Accessed January 11, 2012.

154. Pope TM, West A. Legal briefing: voluntarily stopping eating and drinking. *J Clin Ethics.* 2014;25(1):68-80.

155. Quill TE. Voluntary stopping of eating and drinking (VSED), physician-assisted death (PAD), or neither in the last stage of life? Both should be available as a last resort. *Ann Fam Med.* 2015;13(5):408-409.

156. Ivanovic N, Buche D, Fringer A. Voluntary stopping of eating and drinking at the end of life—a 'systematic search and review' giving insight into an option of hastening death in capacitated adults at the end of life. *BMC Palliat Care.* 2014;13(1):1.

157. Meier CA, Ong TD. To feed or not to feed? A case report and ethical analysis of withholding food and drink in a patient with advanced dementia. *J Pain Symptom Manage.* 2015;50(6):887-890.

158. Palecek EJ, Teno JM, Casarett DJ, Hanson LC, Rhodes RL, Mitchell SL. Comfort feeding only: a proposal to bring clarity to decision-making regarding difficulty with eating for persons with advanced dementia. *J Am Geriatr Soc.* 2010;58(3):580-584.

159. Menzel PT, Chandler-Cramer MC. Advance directives, dementia, and withholding food and water by mouth. *Hastings Cent Rep.* 2014;44(3):23-37.

160. Kirk TW, Mahon MM. National Hospice and Palliative Care Organization (NHPCO) position statement and commentary on the use of palliative sedation in imminently dying terminally ill patients. *J Pain Symptom Manage.* 2010;39(5):914-923.

161. Lux MR, Protus BM, Kimbrel J, Grauer P. A survey of hospice and palliative care physicians regarding palliative sedation practices. *Am J Hosp Palliat Care.* 2015.

162. Maltoni M, Scarpi E, Nanni O. Palliative sedation for intolerable suffering. *Curr Opin Oncol.* 2014;26(4):389-394.

163. Beller EM, van Driel ML, McGregor L, Truong S, Mitchell G. Palliative pharmacological sedation for terminally ill adults. *Cochrane Database Syst Rev.* 2015;1:Cd010206.

164. Maeda I, Morita T, Yamaguchi T, et al. Effect of continuous deep sedation on survival in patients with advanced cancer (J-Proval): a propensity score-weighted analysis of a prospective cohort study. *Lancet Oncol.* 2016;17(1):115-122.

165. Schildmann E, Schildmann J. Palliative sedation therapy: a systematic literature review and critical appraisal of available guidance on indication and decision making. *J Palliat Med.* 2014;17(5):601-611.

166. American Medical Association. Opinion 2.201—Sedation to Unconsciousness in End-of-Life Care. 2008. Accessed June 20, 2016.

167. American Academy of Hospice and Palliative Medicine. Statement on Palliative Sedation. 2014; http://aahpm.org/positions/palliative-sedation. Accessed June 20, 2016.

168. Rousseau P. Palliative sedation in the management of refractory symptoms. *J Support Oncol.* 2004;2(2):181-186.

169. Quill TE, Byock IR. Responding to intractable terminal suffering. *Ann Intern Med.* 2000;133(7):561-562.

170. Salacz M, Weissman D. Fast facts and concepts #106: controlled sedation for refractory suffering—part 1. End-of-Life/Palliative Education Resource Center. 2004; www.eperc.mcw.edu/ff_index.htm. Accessed August 3, 2007.

171. Salacz M, Weissman D. Fast facts and concepts #107: controlled sedation for refractory suffering--part II. End-of-Life/Palliative Education Resource Center. 2004; www.eperc.mcw.edu/ff_index.htm. Accessed August 3, 2007.

172. Cherny N. Palliative sedation (Table—Medications used for palliative sedation in patients with refractory symptoms at the end of life). *UpToDate.* 2017.

173. Yang YT, Curlin FA. Why physicians should oppose assisted suicide. *JAMA.* 2016;315(3):247-248.

174. New York State Task Force on Life and the Law. The ethical debate. *When Death Is Sought.* 1994:77-113.

175. Quill TE, Back AL, Block SD. Responding to patients requesting physician-assisted death: physician involvement at the very end of life. *JAMA.* 2016;315(3):245-246.

176. Snyder L, Sulmasy DP. Physician-assisted suicide. *Ann Intern Med.* 2001;135:209-216.

177. American Nurses Association. Position statement: euthanasia, assisted suicide, and aid in dying. 2013.

178. The Ethics and Humanities Subcommittee of the American Academy of Neurology. Assisted suicide, euthanasia, and the neurologist. *Neurology.* 1998;50(3):596-598.

179. Views on end-of-life medical treatments. 2013. http://www.pewforum.org/2013/11/21/views-on-end-of-life-medical-treatments/.

180. Religious groups' views on end-of-life issues. 2013; http://www.pewforum.org/2013/11/21/religious-groups-views-on-end-of-life-issues/.

181. Foley KM. Competent care for the dying instead of physician-assisted suicide. *N Engl J Med.* 1997;336(1):54-58.

182. *Oregon death with dignity act: 2015 data summary.* 2016.

183. American Medical Women's Association. American Medical Women's Association position paper on aid in dying. 2007; https://www.amwa-doc.org/wp-content/uploads/2013/12/Aid_in_Dying1.pdf Accessed June 4, 2016.

184. California Medical Association. California Medical Association removes opposition to physician aid in dying bill. 2015; http://www.cmanet.org/news/press-detail/?article=california-medical-association-removes. Accessed June 5, 2016.

185. American Academy of Hospice and Palliative Medicine. Statement on physician-assisted dying. 2016. Accessed June 24, 2016.

186. California Natural Death Act, §1 (1976).

187. *Washington v Glucksberg,* 521 US 702 (1997).

188. Gostin LO, Roberts AE. Physician-assisted dying: a turning point? *JAMA.* 2016;315(3):249-250.

189. *Baxter v State,* 224 P3d 1211 (2009).

190. Oregon Death with Dignity Act, §127.805 (1997).

191. *Gonzales v Oregon,* 546 US 243 (2006).

192. Assisted Suicide Funding Restriction Act, 42 USC, §14401 (1997).

193. The Task Force to Improve the Care of Terminally Ill Oregonians. The Oregon death with dignity act: a guidebook for health care professionals. 2008: https://www.ohsu.edu/xd/education/continuing-education/center-for-ethics/ethics-outreach/upload/Oregon-Death-with-Dignity-Act-Guidebook.pdf. Accessed June 3, 2016.

194. American Academy of Hospice and Palliative Medicine. Advisory brief: guidance on responding to requests for physician-assisted dying. 2016.

195. Orentlicher D, Pope TM, Rich BA. Clinical criteria for physician aid in dying. *J Palliat Med.* 2016;19(3):259-262.

196. Steck N, Egger M, Maessen M, Reisch T, Zwahlen M. Euthanasia and assisted suicide in selected European countries and US states: systematic literature review. *Med Care.* 2013;51(10):938-944.

197. Emanuel EJ, Onwuteaka-Philipsen BD, Urwin JW, Cohen J. Attitudes and practices of euthanasia and physician-assisted suicide in the United States, Canada, and Europe. *JAMA.* 2016;316(1):79-90.

198. Washington Death with Dignity Act, Wash Rev Code, §70.245 (2008).

199. Vermont Patient Choice and Control at End of Life Act, §18.113 (2013).

200. California End of Life Option Act, Health and Safety Code, §443 (2016).

201. Van Der Maas PJ, Van Delden JJ, Pijnenborg L, Looman CW. Euthanasia and other medical decisions concerning the end of life. *Lancet.* 1991;338(8768):669-674.

202. Ganzini L, Nelson HD, Schmidt TA, Kraemer DF, Delorit MA, Lee MA. Physicians' experiences with the Oregon Death with Dignity Act. *N Engl J Med.* 2000;342(8):557-563.

203. Pearlman RA, Hsu C, Starks H, et al. Motivations for physician-assisted suicide. *J Gen Intern Med.* 2005;20(3):234-239.

204. Ganzini L, Goy ER, Dobscha SK. Oregonians' reasons for requesting physician aid in dying. *Arch Intern Med.* 2009;169(5):489-492.

205. *Washington State Department of Health 2015 Death with Dignity Act report executive summary.* 2015.

206. Cassell EJ, Rich BA. Intractable end-of-life suffering and the ethics of palliative sedation. *Pain Med.* 2010;11(3):435-438.

207. Gather J, Vollmann J. Physician-assisted suicide of patients with dementia. A medical ethical analysis with a special focus on patient autonomy. *Int J Law Psychiatry.* 2013;36(5-6):444-453.

208. Schuklenk U, van de Vathorst S. Treatment-resistant major depressive disorder and assisted dying: response to comments. *J Med Ethics*. 2015;41(8):589-591.

209. Snijdewind MC, Willems DL, Deliens L, Onwuteaka-Philipsen BD, Chambaere K. A study of the first year of the end-of-life clinic for physician-assisted dying in the Netherlands. *JAMA Intern Med*. 2015;175(10):1633-1640.

210. Thienpont L, Verhofstadt M, Van Loon T, Distelmans W, Audenaert K, De Deyn PP. Euthanasia requests, procedures and outcomes for 100 Belgian patients suffering from psychiatric disorders: a retrospective, descriptive study. *BMJ Open*. 2015;5(7):e007454.

211. Menzel PT, Steinbock B. Advance directives, dementia, and physician-assisted death. *J Law Med Ethics*. 2013;41(2):484-500.

212. Kim SY, De Vries RG, Peteet JR. Euthanasia and assisted suicide of patients with psychiatric disorders in the Netherlands 2011 to 2014. *JAMA Psychiatry*. 2016;73(4):362-368.

213. Duffy OA. The Supreme Court of Canada ruling on physician-assisted death: implications for psychiatry in Canada. *Canadian journal of psychiatry. Revue canadienne de psychiatrie*. 2015;60(12):591-596.

214. Dan B, Fonteyne C, de Clety SC. Self-requested euthanasia for children in Belgium. *Lancet*. 2014;383(9918):671-672.

215. van der Heide A, Onwuteaka-Philipsen BD, Rurup ML, et al. End-of-life practices in the Netherlands under the Euthanasia Act. *N Engl J Med*. 2007;356(19):1957-1965.

216. ten Cate K, van de Vathorst S, Onwuteaka-Philipsen BD, van der Heide A. End-of-life decisions for children under 1 year of age in the Netherlands: decreased frequency of administration of drugs to deliberately hasten death. *J Med Ethics*. 2015;41(10):795-798.

217. Verhagen E, Sauer PJ. The Groningen protocol—euthanasia in severely ill newborns. *N Engl J Med*. 2005;352(10):959-962.

218. Willems DL, Verhagen AA, van Wijlick E. Infants' best interests in end-of-life care for newborns. *Pediatrics*. 2014;134(4):e1163-1168.

219. American Academy of Hospice and Palliative Medicine. Advisory Brief: Guidance on Responding to Requests for Physician-Assisted Dying. http://aahpm.org/positions/padbrief. Accessed May 31, 2017.

220. American Academy of Hospice and Palliative Medicine. Statement on Physician-Assisted Dying. 2016; http://aahpm.org/positions/pad. Accessed May 31, 2017.

221. Nelson JL. Internal organs, integral selves, and good communities: opt-out organ procurement policies and the 'separateness of persons'. *Theor Med Bioeth*. 2011;32(5):289-300.

222. Prommer E. Organ donation and palliative care: can palliative care make a difference? *J Palliat Med*. 2014;17(3):368-371.

223. Rady MY, Verheijde JL, McGregor J. Organ donation after circulatory death: the forgotten donor? *Crit Care*. 2006;10(5):166.

224. Kesselring A, Kainz M, Kiss A. Traumatic memories of relatives regarding brain death, request for organ donation and interactions with professionals in the ICU. *Am J Transplant*. 2007;7(1):211-217.

225. Hospice & Palliative Nurses Association. HPNA position statement: the role of palliative care in organ and tissue donation. 2013.

226. Services USDoHaH. Advisory commmittee on organ transplantation. Accessed May 4, 2016.

227. Arnold RM. Fast facts and concepts #79: discussing organ donation with families. 2006; www.aahpm.org/cgi-bin/wkcgi/view?status=A%20&search=155&id=390&offset=0&limit=258. Accessed August 3, 2007.

228. Arnold RM, Siminoff LA, Frader JE. Ethical issues in organ procurement: a review for intensivists. *Crit Care Clin*. 1996;12(1):29-48.

229. Siminoff LA, Arnold RM, Caplan AL, Virnig BA, Seltzer DL. Public policy governing organ and tissue procurement in the United States. Results from the National Organ and Tissue Procurement Study. *Ann Intern Med.* 1995;123(1):10-17.

230. Siminoff LA, Gordon N, Hewlett J, Arnold RM. Factors influencing families' consent for donation of solid organs for transplantation. *JAMA.* 2001;286(1):71-77.

231. Institute of Medicine. *Dying in America: Improving Quality and Honoring Individual Preferences Near the End of Life.* Washington, DC: The Natinoal Academies Press; 2015.

232. Casarett D, Karlawish J, Morales K, Crowley R, Mirsch T, Asch DA. Improving the use of hospice services in nursing homes: a randomized controlled trial. *JAMA.* 2005;294(2):211-217.

233. Oliver DP, Washington K, Kruse RL, Albright DL, Lewis A, Demiris G. Hospice family members' perceptions of and experiences with end-of-life care in the nursing home. *J Am Med Dir Assoc.* 2014;15(10):744-750.

234. Meyers JL, Moore C, McGrory A, Sparr J, Ahern M. Physician orders for life-sustaining treatment form: honoring end-of-life directives for nursing home residents. *J Gerontol Nurs.* 2004;30(9):37-46.

235. Zheng NT, Mukamel DB, Friedman B, Caprio TV, Temkin-Greener H. The effect of hospice on hospitalizations of nursing home residents. *J Am Med Dir Assoc.* 2015;16(2):155-159.

236. Lester PE, Stefanacci RG, Feuerman M. Prevalence and description of palliative care in US nursing homes: a descriptive study. *Am J Hosp Palliat Care.* 2016;33(2):171-177.

237. Gozalo P, Plotzke M, Mor V, Miller SC, Teno JM. Changes in Medicare costs with the growth of hospice care in nursing homes. *N Engl J Med.* 2015;372(19):1823-1831.

238. Aldridge MD, Schlesinger M, Barry CL, et al. National hospice survey results: for-profit status, community engagement, and service. *JAMA Intern Med.* 2014;174(4):500-506.

239. Unroe KT, Sachs GA, Dennis ME, et al. Hospice use among nursing home and non-nursing home patients. *J Gen Intern Med.* 2015;30(2):193-198.

240. Cloyes KG, Rosenkranz SJ, Berry PH, et al. Essential elements of an effective prison hospice program. *Am J Hosp Palliat Care.* 2016;33(4):390-402.

241. The National Prison Hospice Association. www.npha.org. Accessed June 3, 2016.

242. Schinka JA, Curtiss G, Leventhal K, Bossarte RM, Lapcevic W, Casey R. Predictors of mortality in older homeless veterans. *J Gerontol B Psychol Sci Soc Sci.* 2016.

243. Podymow T, Turnbull J, Coyle D. Shelter-based palliative care for the homeless terminally ill. *Palliat Med.* 2006;20(2):81-86.

244. Epstein EG, Hamric AB. Moral distress, moral residue, and the crescendo effect. *J Clin Ethics.* 2009;20(4):330-342.

245. Corley MC. Nurse moral distress: a proposed theory and research agenda. *Nurs Ethics.* 2002;9(6):636-650.

246. Helft PR, Bledsoe PD, Hancock M, Wocial LD. Facilitated ethics conversations: a novel program for managing moral distress in bedside nursing staff. *JONA'S Healthcare Law Ethics Reg.* 2009;11(1):27-33.

247. American Association of Critical Care Nurses. 4 a's to rise above moral distress. http://www.aacn.org/WD/Practice/Content/ethic-moral.pcms?menu=Practice Accessed June 30, 2015.

248. Dudzinski DM. Navigating moral distress using the moral distress map. *J Med Ethics.* 2016;42(5):321-324.

249. Pavlish C, Brown-Saltzman K, So L, Wong J. SUPPORT: an evidence-based model for leaders addressing moral distress. *J Nurs Admin.* 2016;46(6):313-320.

250. Vig EK, Foglia MB. The steak dinner—a professional boundary crossing. *J Pain Symptom Manage.* 2014;48(3):483-487.

251. Farber NJ, Novack DH, O'Brien MK. Love, boundaries, and the patient-physician relationship. *Arch Intern Med.* 1997;157(20):2291-2294.

252. Reeh PW, Steen KH. Tissue acidosis in nociception and pain. *Prog. Brain Res.* 1996;113:143-151.

253. Aktas A, Walsh D. Methodological challenges in supportive and palliative care cancer research. *Semin Oncol.* 2011;38(3):460-466.

254. Casarett D. Ethical considerations in end-of-life care and research. *J Palliat Med.* 2005;8 Suppl 1:S148-160.

255. Beecher HK. Ethics and clinical research. 1966. *Bull World Health Organ.* 2001;79(4):367-372.

256. Kristjanson LJ, Hanson EJ, Balneaves L. Research in palliative care populations: ethical issues. *J Palliat Care.* 1994;10(3):10-15.

257. Tan H, Wilson A, Olver I, Barton C. Recruiting palliative patients for a large qualitative study: some ethical considerations and staff dilemmas. *Explore (NY).* 2010;6(3):159-165.

258. Appelbaum PS, Roth LH, Lidz CW, Benson P, Winslade W. False hopes and best data: consent to research and the therapeutic misconception. *Hastings Cent Rep.* 1987;17(2):20-24.

259. Coleman C, Menikoff J, Goldner J, Dubler N. *The Ethics and Regulation of Research with Human Subjects.* Matthew Bender; 2005.

260. Criteria for IRB approval of research. To be codified at 45 CFR §46.111. *Fed Registr.* 2005.

261. General requirements for informed consent. To be codified at 45 CFR §46.116. *Fed Registr.* 2005.

262. Casarett DJ, Karlawish JH. Are special ethical guidelines needed for palliative care research? *J Pain Symptom Manage.* 2000;20(2):130-139.

263. Sweet L, Adamis D, Meagher DJ, et al. Ethical challenges and solutions regarding delirium studies in palliative care. *J Pain Symptom Manage.* 2014;48(2):259-271.

264. Slaughter S, Cole D, Jennings E, Reimer MA. Consent and assent to participate in research from people with dementia. *Nurs Ethics.* 2007;14(1):27-40.

265. American Academy of Hospice and Palliative Medicine. Statement on Palliative Care Research. 2014; http://aahpm.org/positions/research-ethics. Accessed May 31, 2017.

266. *Superintendent of Belchertown State School v Saikewicz,* 370 NE2d 417, 431 (Mass. 1977).

267. *State of Georgia v. McAfee,* 259 579(Ga. 1989).

268. Ahronheim JC, Mulvihill M. Refusal of tube feeding as seen from a patient advocacy organization: a comparison with landmark court cases. *J Am Geriatr Soc.* 1991;39(11):1124-1127.

269. Miles SH. Informed demand for "non-beneficial" medical treatment. *N Engl J Med.* 1991;325(7):512-515.

270. *In re Quinlan,* 355 A2d 647 (NJ 1976).

271. Kinney HC, Korein J, Panigrahy A, Dikkes P, Goode R. Neuropathological findings in the brain of Karen Ann Quinlan. The role of the thalamus in the persistent vegetative state. *N Engl J Med.* 1994;330(21):1469-1475.

272. *In the Matter of Spring,* 405 NE2d 115,121 (Mass. 1980).

273. *matter of Storar,* 106 880(Misc.2d 1980).

274. Wynn S. Decisions by surrogates: an overview of surrogate consent laws in the United States. *Bifocal.* 2014;36(1).

275. *Barber v Superior Court,* 147 CA Rptr 484 (Ct App 1983).

276. *In re Conroy,* 486 A2d 1209 (NY 1985).

277. NSJA, 27G 52, §2a (2013).

278. Price DM, Armstrong PW. New Jersey's "Granny Doe" squad: arguments about mechanisms for protection of vulnerable patients. *Law Med Health Care.* 1989;17(3):255-263.

279. *In the Matter of Claire C. Conroy,* 98 321(N.J. 1985).

280. *Bouvia v Superior Court,* 225 Cal. Rptr. 297 (Ct App 1986).

281. *In the Matter of Baby K,* 16 F3d 590 (4th Cir. 1993).

282. Hall MA, Bobinski MA, Orentlicher D. *Medical Liability and Treatment Relationships.* 2nd ed. New York, NY: Aspen Publishers, Inc.; 2008.

283. Burt RA. The Supreme Court speaks--not assisted suicide but a constitutional right to palliative care. *N Engl J Med.* 1997;337(17):1234-1236.

284. *In re Guardianship of Schiavo,* 780 So2d 176, 180 (FL App. Ct. 2001).

285. Richey W, Feldmann L. Who speaks for Terri Schiavo? *The Christian Science Monitor.* 2005. http://www.csmonitor.com/2005/0323/p01s04-ussc.html. Accessed June 16, 2016.

286. University of Miami Ethics Programs, Shepard Broad Law Center at Nova Southeastern University. Key events in the case of Theresa Marie Schiavo. http://www6.miami.edu/ethics/schiavo/timeline.htm. Accessed January 12, 2012.

287. *Bush v Schiavo,* 885 So2d 321 (FL 2004).

288. Fine RL. From Quinlan to Schiavo: medical, ethical, and legal issues in severe brain injury. *Proceedings (Baylor University. Medical Center).* 2005;18(4):303-310.

289. Bernat JL. Chronic disorders of consciousness. *Lancet.* 2006;367(9517):1181-1192.

290. Annas GJ. "Culture of life" politics at the bedside--the case of Terri Schiavo. *N Engl J Med.* 2005;352(16):1710-1715.

291. Cerminara K, Goodman K. Schiavo Timeline, Part 1-3. http://www.miami.edu/index.php/ethics/projects/schiavo/schiavo_timeline/. Accessed June 15, 2016.

292. Breault JL. DNR, DNAR, or AND? Is language important? *Ochsner J.* 2011;11(4)302-306.

293. Stone K, Papadopoulos I, Kelly D. Establishing hospice care for prison populations: an integrative review assessing the UK and USA perspective. *Palliat Med.* Oct 12 2011.

294. Maull FW. Issues in prison hospice: toward a model for the delivery of hospice care in a correctional setting. *Hosp J.* 1998;13(4):57-82.

295. Seidlitz A. Doing "family" in a women's hospice. *NPHA News.* 1999;6:8-9.

296. Hoffman HC, Dickinson GE. Characteristics of prison hospice programs in the United States. *Am J Hosp Palliat Care.* Jun 2011;28(4):245-252.

297. US Department of Housing and Urban Development. The 2015 Annual Homeless Assessment Report (AHAR) to Congress. Washington, DC: US Department of Housing and Urban Development; 2015. https://www.hudexchange.info/resources/documents/2015-AHAR-Part-1.pdf. Accessed August 8, 2017.

Index